The Burden of Respiratory Syncytial Virus Infection in the Young

Edited by Bernhard Resch

Published in London, United Kingdom

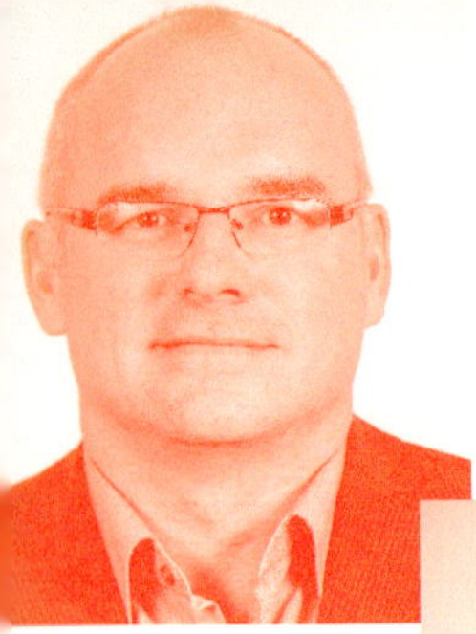
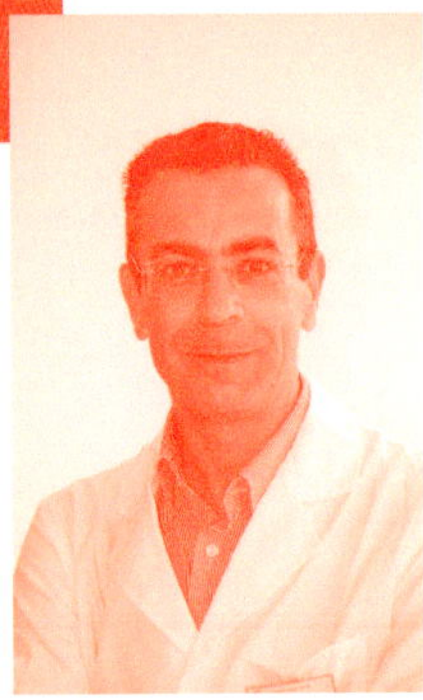
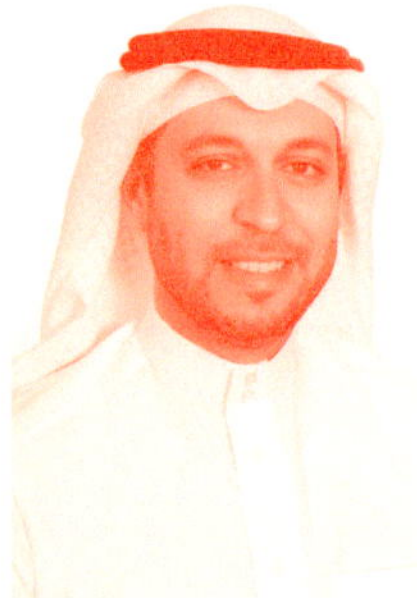
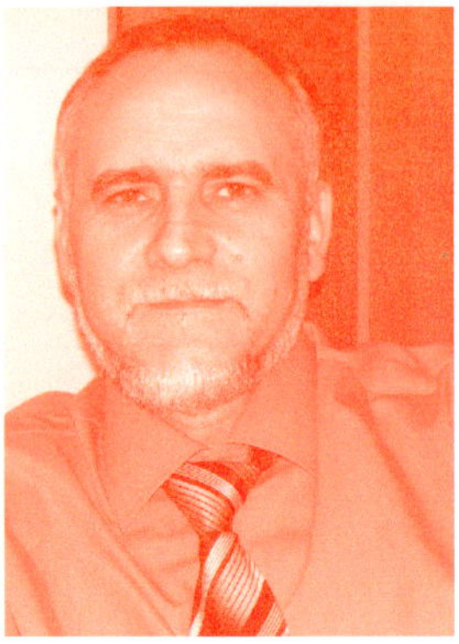
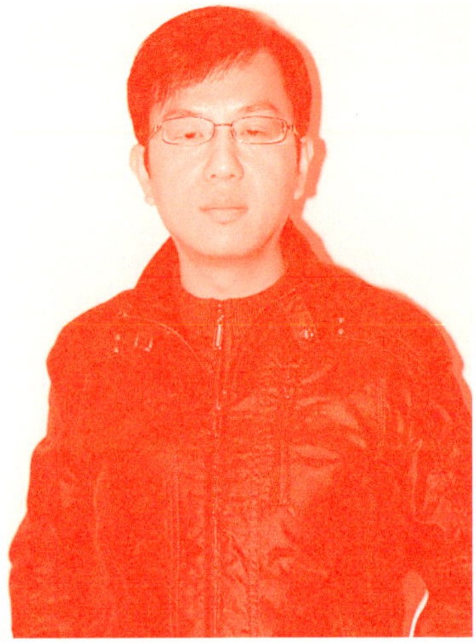
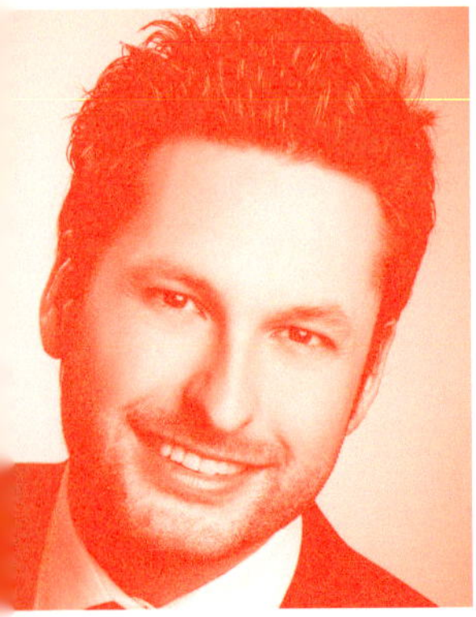
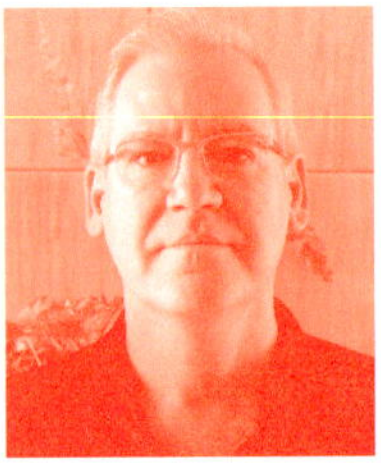

IntechOpen

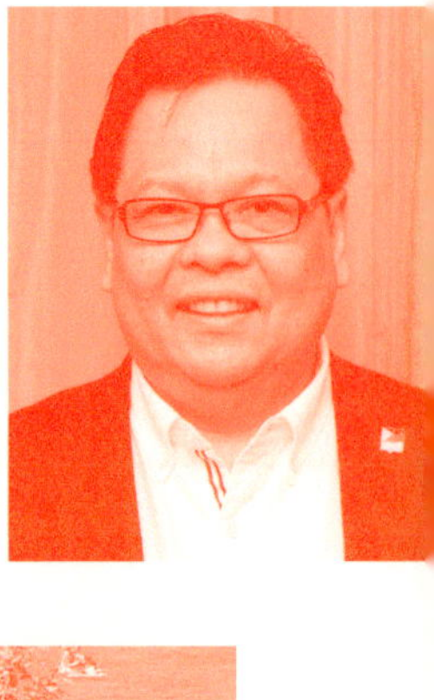
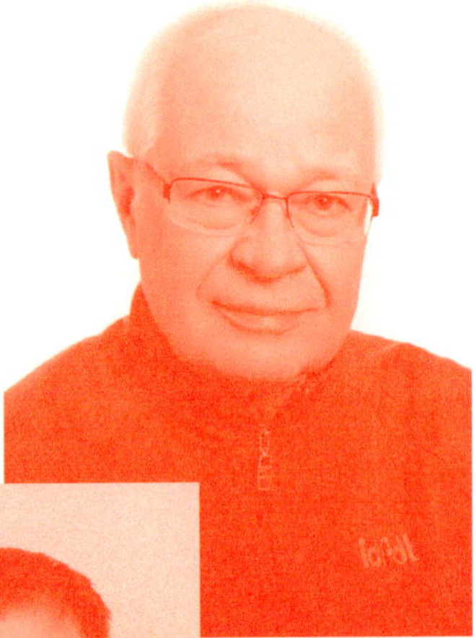
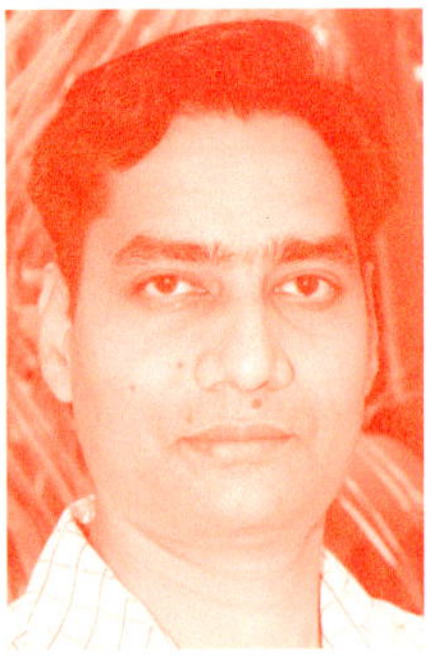
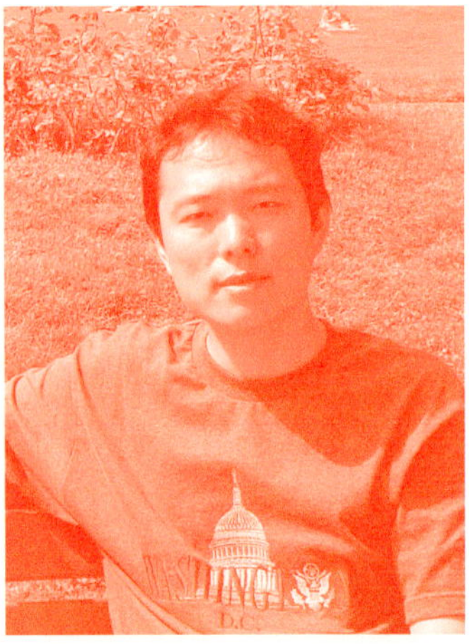
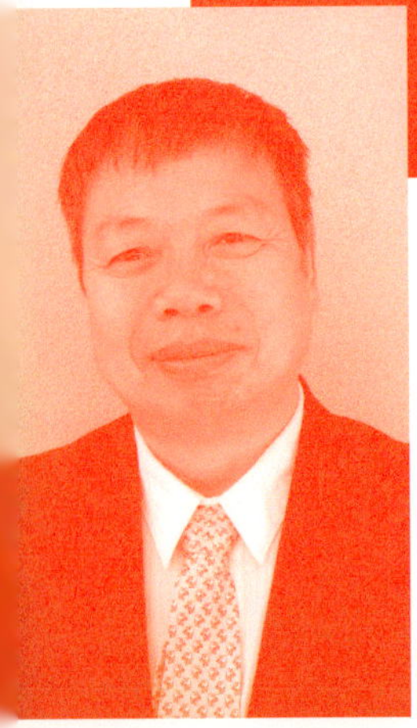
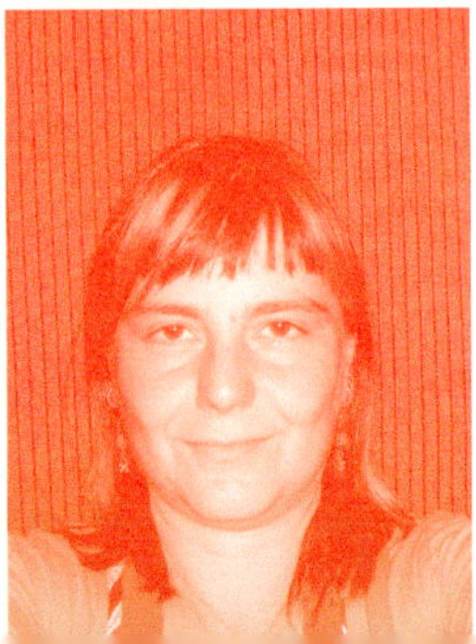

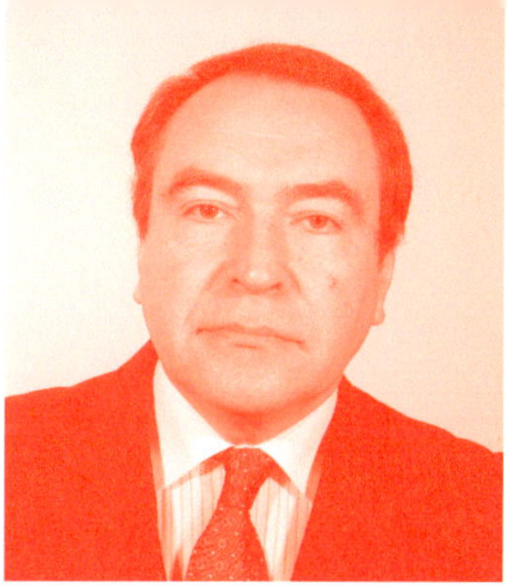
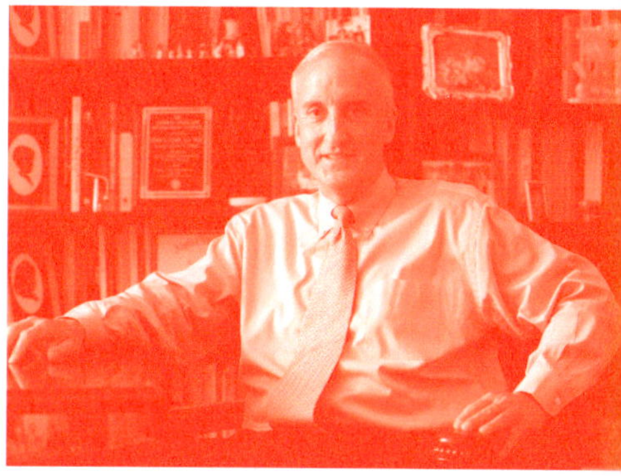
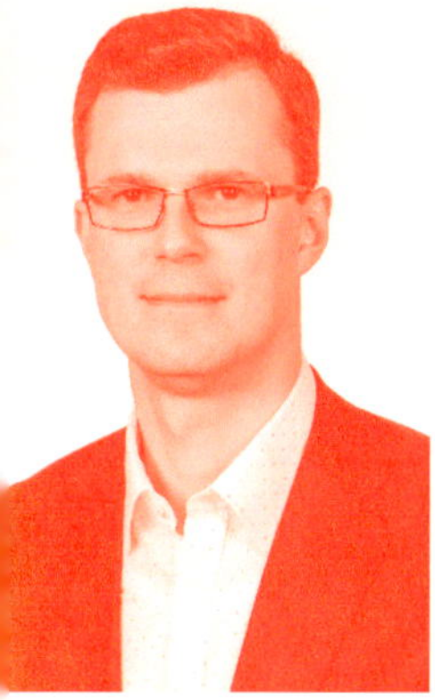
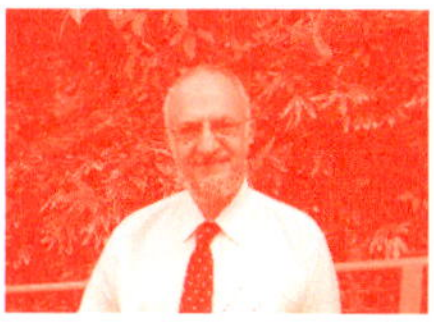
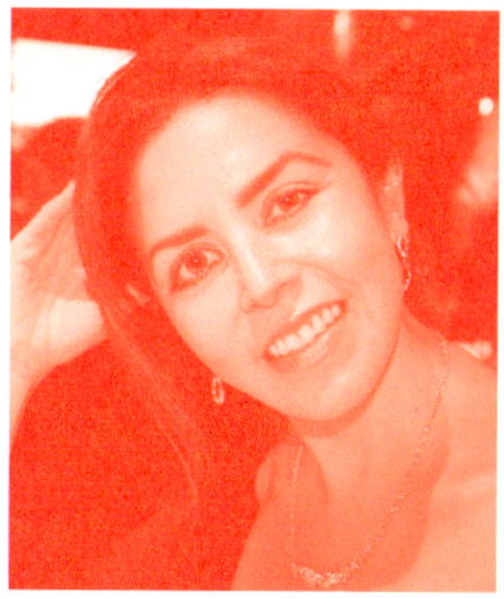

Supporting open minds since 2005

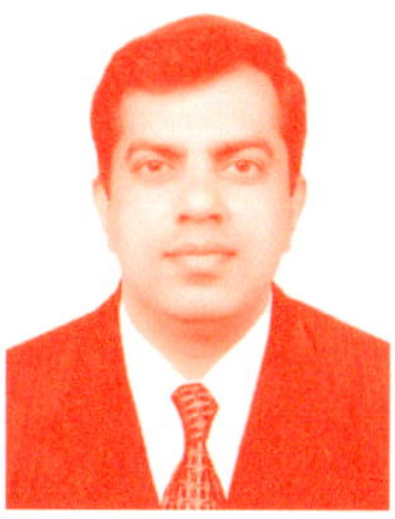
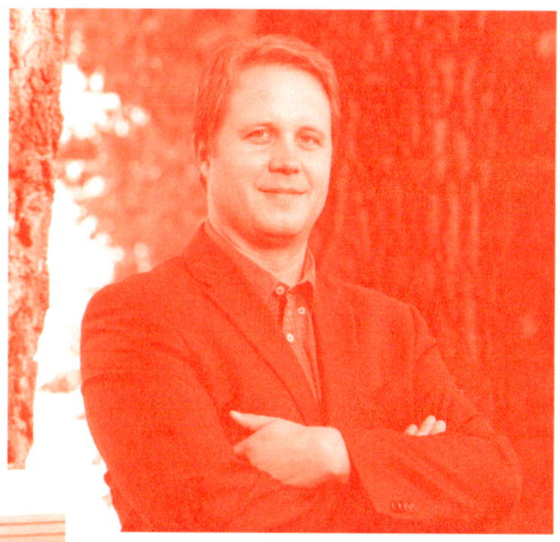
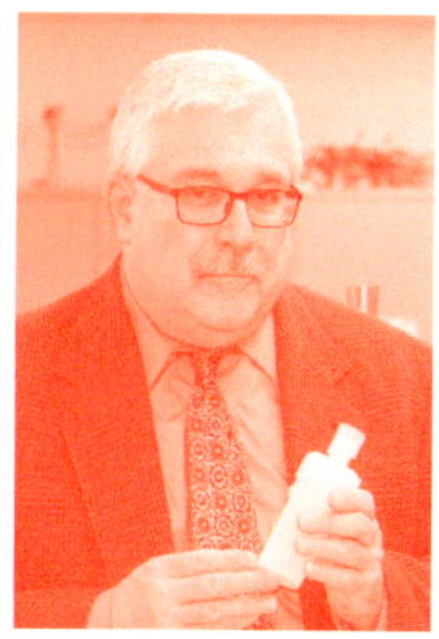
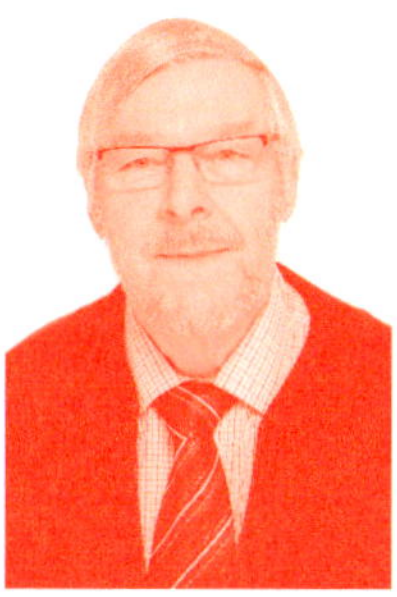
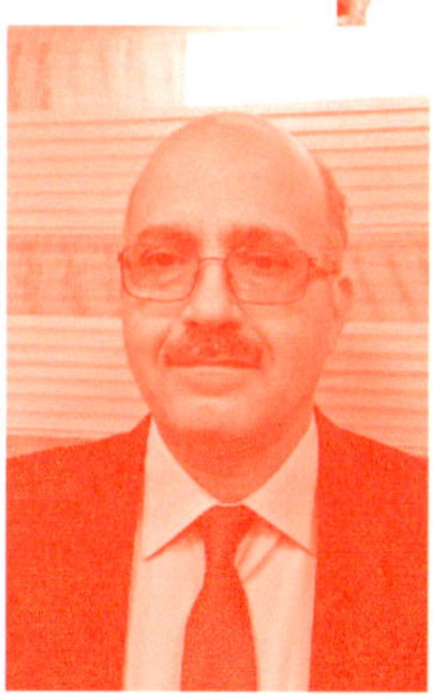
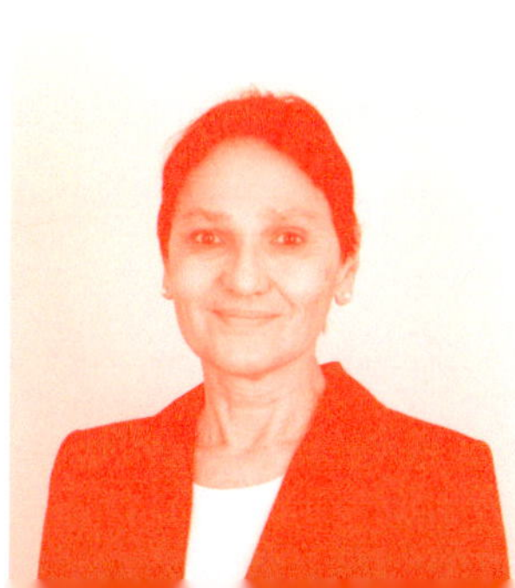
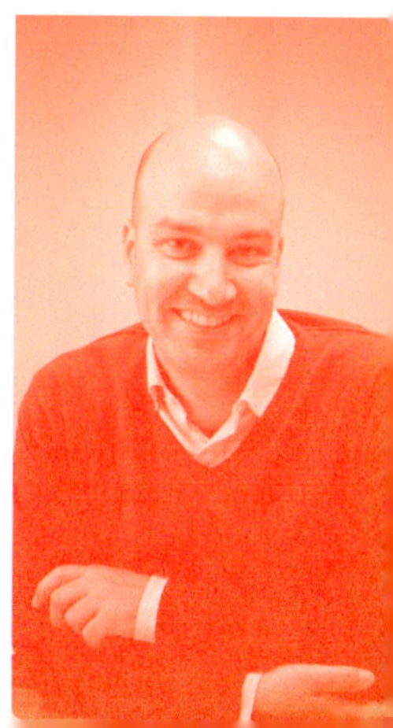

The Burden of Respiratory Syncytial Virus Infection in the Young
http://dx.doi.org/10.5772/intechopen.78206
Edited by Bernhard Resch

Contributors
Muhammad Shafique, Muhammad Zahoor, Muhammad Imran Arshad, Bilal Aslam, Abu Baker Siddique, Muhammad Hidayat Rasool, Muhammad Usman Qamar, Muhammad Usman, Bosco Paes, Xavier Carbonell-Estrany, Barry Rodgers-Gray, Fariba Rezaee, Debra Linfield, Maja Daurach, Julian Legg

Notice
Statements and opinions expressed in the chapters are these of the individual contributors and not necessarily those of the editors or publisher. No responsibility is accepted for the accuracy of information contained in the published chapters. The publisher assumes no responsibility for any damage or injury to persons or property arising out of the use of any materials, instructions, methods or ideas contained in the book.

First published in London, United Kingdom, 2019 by IntechOpen
IntechOpen is the global imprint of INTECHOPEN LIMITED, registered in England and Wales, registration number: 11086078, 7th floor, 10 Lower Thames Street, London, EC3R 6AF, United Kingdom
Printed in Croatia

British Library Cataloguing-in-Publication Data
A catalogue record for this book is available from the British Library

Additional hard and PDF copies can be obtained from orders@intechopen.com

The Burden of Respiratory Syncytial Virus Infection in the Young
Edited by Bernhard Resch
p. cm.
Print ISBN 978-1-78984-642-3
Online ISBN 978-1-78984-643-0
eBook (PDF) ISBN 978-1-83962-252-6

For EU product safety concerns:
IN TECH d.o.o., Prolaz Marije Krucifikse Kozulić 3, 51000 Rijeka, Croatia, info@intechopen.com or visit our website at intechopen.com.

Meet the editor

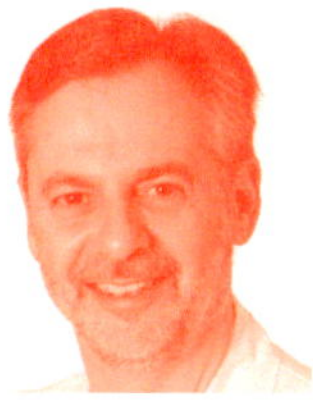

Born in Graz, Austria, Prof. Bernhard Resch received his medical degree at the University of Graz in 1988. Following post-doctoral studies at the Division of Neonatology and the Department of Pediatric Surgery at the University Hospital Graz, he became consultant of Pediatrics in 1997 and consultant of Neonatal and Pediatric Intensive Care Medicine in 2000. Since 2004 he has served as Associate Professor of Pediatrics, and since 2008 he has served as head of the research unit of Neonatal Infectious Diseases and Epidemiology of the Medical University Graz. In 2012 he graduated as Professor of Pediatrics and in 2013 he became Deputy Head of the Division of Neonatology of the Medical University of Graz. His main research fields include neonatal infectious diseases and periventricular leukomalacia of the preterm infant.

He is a member of the Austrian Society of Pediatrics and Adolescent Medicine (ÖGKJ), the European Society of Pediatric Infectious Diseases (ESPID), and the Austrian Society of Perinatal Medicine (ÖGPPM; president from 2012 to 2014). He was also head of the Austrian Working Group of Neonatology and Pediatric Intensive Care Medicine from 2009 to 2011. Dr. Resch is an associate and academic editor of several SCI-listed journals including *BMC Infectious Diseases*, *Medicine*, and *Frontiers in Pediatrics*. Dr. Resch is married and has four children aged 19 to 29 years.

Contents

Preface

Respiratory syncytial virus (RSV) causes seasonal epidemics during the winter and wet seasons, particularly in young children. Of the children infected with RSV, 70%–90% are diagnosed with bronchiolitis and hospitalized because they need supplemental oxygen. Approximately 1% of healthy young infants are hospitalized during the first RSV season due to severe lower respiratory tract infection. Three to ten times higher rates of RSV have been reported in high-risk populations, including preterm infants; those with bronchopulmonary dysplasia; infants and children with congenital heart disease, cystic fibrosis, congenital diaphragmatic hernia, neuromuscular disease, or Down syndrome; and immunocompromised infants. After two RSV seasons and three years of age, nearly 100% of children have experienced an RSV infection or have antibodies against RSV. However, despite neutralizing antibodies, recurrent infections do occur. Severity of disease, though, decreases as children become older.

For the last 20 years, palivizumab has been used for immunoprophylaxis of RSV infections. It is a monoclonal antibody that binds to the F-glycoprotein that is 95% identical between the G- and F-receptor and thus works against RSV types A and B. Palivizumab is given to high-risk infants only, hence the burden of RSV diseases continues to grow and a vaccine is urgently needed.

Following a fatal vaccine trial in the early 1960s that led to two deaths, many efforts to develop a safe vaccine have been undertaken. This book covers the problems the young RSV patient faces and provides data on the most recent vaccine progresses and new monoclonal antibodies. It is our hope that this volume will open up new avenues to future tools in RSV prophylaxis.

Palivizumab (Synagis®, MedImmune, Inc., USA) is a humanized monoclonal antibody that provides immunoprophylaxis against respiratory syncytial virus (RSV). RSV causes seasonal epidemics (winter or wet-season) of serious lower respiratory tract infections in young infants with subsequent increased frequency of recurrent wheezing during early childhood. Two large, double-blind, placebo-controlled trials including infants at high risk for severe RSV infection showed significant reduction of RSV-related hospitalizations: a 55% reduction in 1502 infants with prematurity and/or bronchopulmonary dysplasia and a 45% reduction in 1287 infants with hemodynamically significant congenital heart disease. Palivizumab proved to be as safe as an intramuscular injection of 15 mg/kg every 30 days for

5 months according to local epidemiology. Recent data suggest further benefits for palivizumab prophylaxis by reduction of recurrent post-RSV wheezing.

Bernhard Resch, MD
Professor,
Division of Neonatology,
Department of Pediatrics and Adolescent Medicine,
Medical University of Graz,
Graz, Austria

Section 1

RSV Immunology

Chapter 1

Disease Severity in Respiratory Syncytial Virus Infection: Role of Viral and Host Factors

Julian P. Legg

Abstract

Respiratory syncytial virus (RSV) is not only a major cause of severe lower respiratory tract infection (LRTI) in infancy but is increasingly recognised as an important pathogen in later life. RSV infection is associated with a wide spectrum of disease ranging from asymptomatic infection to life-threatening bronchiolitis and pneumonia. Research has demonstrated that there exists a complex interplay between viral and host factors that determines the severity of disease following RSV infection. Several factors determine RSV virulence including the infective properties of individual strains and viral load (VL). Disease outcome from RSV infection is also impacted considerably by a variety of host factors with the host immune response increasingly recognised as pivotal. This chapter outlines our current understanding of these factors and provides an oversight of their relative importance.

Keywords: respiratory syncytial virus, disease severity, viral load, immunology, genotype

1. Introduction

Respiratory syncytial virus (RSV) has long been recognised as a cause of severe lower respiratory tract infection (LRTI) in early childhood with increasing evidence of its role as an important pathogen in later life [1]. RSV has many intriguing features including its worldwide distribution, its capacity to cause severe disease in early childhood and its extended impact on respiratory health [2]. Consequently, RSV has been the focus of comprehensive study including host and viral determinants of disease severity.

Serologic data has demonstrated that a high proportion of children (between 50 and 70%) will be infected with RSV in the first year of life [3, 4]. Asymptomatic infection is infrequent during infancy with most infants developing clinical features of an upper respiratory tract infection alone [5]. Following an initial prodromal URTI phase, 25–40% of those infected will progress to develop signs and symptoms of bronchiolitis with tachypnoea and chest recession [5]. Bronchiolitis is usually a mild illness in most infants, but a small proportion (2–3%) will develop severe bronchiolitis necessitating hospitalisation [6]. It has been estimated that nearly 33.8 million new cases of RSV-associated LRTI occur worldwide in children under 5 years of age leading to approximately 3.4 million hospitalizations annually [7]. Mortality from RSV infection in developed countries is rare during infancy although there are an estimated 66,000 and 239,000 yearly deaths in children younger than 5 in the developing world [7, 8].

The major clinical manifestation of RSV in older children and adults is upper respiratory tract illness (rhinitis and acute otitis media) although symptoms tend to last longer and there is an increased incidence of cough and wheeze compared to other respiratory viral infections [9, 10]. Immunity following RSV infection is only effective for a matter of months before the individual is once again susceptible to reinfection [11]. Consequently, reinfection occurs throughout life. LRTI is unusual although RSV accounts for a significant percentage (>4%) of community-acquired pneumonias during epidemics [12]. Elderly adults have an increased risk of lower respiratory tract involvement, with 30–40% of patients having auscultatory findings on examination of the chest [13].

RSV is evidently associated with a wide spectrum of disease which has led to significant interest into those factors that determine the nature of the clinical response to infection. Host, viral and geographical factors interact to dictate the clinical outcome of any viral infection. The viral and host factors that influence the human response to RSV infection are the focus of this chapter.

2. Viral factors

2.1 The virus

Respiratory syncytial virus is a medium-sized (120–300 nm), enveloped, single-stranded RNA virus of the *Paramyxoviridae* family that is a ubiquitous pathogen in all age groups. In 1956, it was first isolated from upper respiratory tract specimens collected from a chimpanzee with coryza [14], being subsequently recovered from two children in Baltimore with lower respiratory tract disease [15]. Its identification as a principal cause of bronchiolitis took a further 4 years [16].

2.2 Viral genome and proteins

RSV has a negative polarity RNA genome composed of 15,000 nucleotides with an estimated weight of 500 kDa. The non-segmented RNA genome encodes 10 units from which 11 proteins are translated. The RSV nucleocapsid core consists of the viral genomic RNA wrapped with N protein (called the N-RNA template), the major viral phosphoprotein, encoded by the P gene and the major subunit of the RNA-dependent RNA polymerase, encoded by the L gene. The genome also encodes for two matrix proteins. The first matrix protein, M, is essential for RSV replication and passaging and plays a central role in virus assembly. The second matrix protein, M2, is localised within the nucleocapsid and has an essential role in the production of complete mRNA during replication. The NS1 and NS2 gene sequences encode for the so-called nonstructural proteins which have been shown to have multiple functions including abrogation of the cellular antiviral response and induction of interferon (IFN) transcription.

Three surface proteins are also encoded within the RSV genome, the fusion (F) protein, the G attachment (G) protein and the small hydrophobic (SH) protein. The F protein plays a central role in virus entry. It mediates fusion between the viral and cellular membrane, thereby allowing the nucleocapsid to enter the cytoplasm of the host cell. The G protein is essential for initial RSV attachment and interaction with the host cell and is important for in vivo replication. The SH protein is a short integral membrane protein that is not essential for RSV replication in cell culture but is involved to some degree in RSV survival in vivo.

2.3 Viral load

The estimation of viral load (VL) has proved invaluable for predicting disease outcome in viral infections such as hepatitis C [17] and HIV [18]. The relationship between the quantity of RSV in respiratory tract specimens and disease severity has been the focus of multiple studies over the last 30 years. There has been significant variability in study findings to date, with some identifying a positive correlation between viral load and severity [19–21], while others have found no significant correlation [22, 23] or an inverse relationship [24]. These disparate outcomes are likely related to the variable nature of the studies with significant differences in age range, enrolment criteria, quantification techniques (plaque assay vs. PCR) and timing of sample collection. The majority of studies have evaluated VL in hospitalised children only and at a single time point.

A number of recent studies have investigated the dynamics of viral load through the analysis of sequential specimens collected during the course of the illness. Garcia-Maurino et al. studied 150 children <2 years of age (39 outpatients and 111 inpatients) over 2 successive winters [25]. Children who required hospitalisation had significantly lower VLs assessed using quantitative PCR on nasal swabs. Sequential VL evaluation (only evaluated in those hospitalised) demonstrated higher initial VLs and a faster VL decline in those requiring ward care only compared to those requiring PICU care. These findings are consistent with the results from a smaller study of 33 infants hospitalised with RSV bronchiolitis using nasosorption sampling of the upper airway [26]. Faster viral clearance was also associated with milder disease and a shorter length of stay in 219 children in Boston with RSV infection whose upper airway VL was assessed using plaque assay [27]. However, by contrast, higher VLs on day 3 of admission were associated with increased disease severity requiring PICU admission.

Studies to date highlight the complexity of the interaction between VL and disease severity. Further studies are required to clarify this relationship and should ideally analyse sequential specimens for changes in viral load in a tightly defined cohort of children and include both hospitalised and community infants with mild disease.

2.4 Genetic and antigenic variability

Through the application of monoclonal antibody technology, two major antigenic groups of RSV have been identified—the A and B subgroups [28]. Epidemiological studies have revealed that these groups have existed for over 40 years and have a worldwide distribution [28]. Both groups appear to circulate concurrently with geographical and temporal clustering frequently reported [29, 30]. The prevalence of each subgroup follows an irregular, alternating pattern with subgroup A predominating in most analyses [29]. The link between the major antigenic groups of RSV and disease severity is unclear. RSV-A has been associated with a more severe disease course in a number of studies [31–33], while others have identified no difference between the subgroups [34–37] or increased severity due to infection with RSV-B [38, 39]. While these inconsistent findings could result from differences in study design and geography, the presence of varying RSV genotypes is likely to be a significant confounding factor.

The RSV genome demonstrates significantly more variability than previously understood [1].

The G protein has been demonstrated as the greatest source of intragroup variability with nucleotide differences of up to 20% [40]. These differences reside predominantly within two variable regions that flank a relatively conserved central ectodomain of the G protein gene.

The single-stranded, non-segmented nature of the RSV genome precludes the genetic rearrangements that typify the dramatic antigenic shifts of the influenza virus [41]. However, there is a considerable potential for genomic mutation given the inability of RNA polymerase to proof-read during replication of the genome. This provides an opportunity for antigenic drift to occur under the influence of selective pressures from the environment. The current variability of the G protein between RSV strains may therefore be explained by the progressive accumulation of change together with survival and extinction of particular genotypes [42].

Prior to whole-genome sequencing, genetic studies have assessed strain variability within the two major groups primarily through analysis of the G protein gene [42, 43]. Subsequent phylogenetic analyses have identified multiple lineages within both group A and group B viruses with marked similarities observed between strains from different locations and time periods [29, 42, 44]. This has led to the recent subclassification of RSV into 14 RSV-A genotypes and 24 RSV-B genotypes [45]. Several distinct RSV strains appear to cocirculate within an individual community during each annual epidemic with the predominant strain varying year to year [44, 46]. Multiple elements appear to determine prevailing annual strains including herd and maternal immunity, changes in social contacts and migration as well as viral factors [29, 47–49].

RSV's capacity for genomic mutation is exemplified by the emergence of two novel genotypes, RSV-B BA and RSV-A ON1 genotypes. In 1999, the BA genotype was first detected in Buenos Aires, Argentina [50], and has since spread gradually and sequentially throughout the world [51], becoming the predominant group B genotype, and even replacing all previous circulating RSV-B genotypes in some regions [52, 53]. Subsequently, the RSV-A genotype ON1 was identified in Ontario, Canada, in 2010 [54] and has rapidly spread worldwide [55]. Both genotypes demonstrate a 60–72 base pair duplication in the G protein gene which may change the antigenic properties of the protein enabling evasion of the host immune response [50, 56].

The possibility that distinct RSV genotypes may have differing virulence has led to several studies in this area. Much interest has concerned the possible association of the ON1 genotype with less severe disease. Panayiotou et al. first described this association in 99 children <2 years of age hospitalised with a RSV respiratory tract infection over 3 successive Cypriot winters [39]. The ON1 genotype was associated with significantly milder illness (as determined by a clinical severity score) than either GA1 (RSV-A) or BA (RSV-B) genotypes. This finding has also been observed in a number of subsequent studies including a recent study of 329 infants with a clinical diagnosis of bronchiolitis and infected with RSV alone [57, 58]. Infants with the NA1 genotype had a milder clinical course both in terms of clinical severity scores and need for admission to PICU. Conversely, other studies have reported a similar clinical course with different genotypes [36, 59] or that genotype ON1 was associated with more severe disease in a group of Vietnamese children hospitalised with signs of LRTI [60].

Once again, the lack of a consistent association between genotype and disease severity is presumably due to variable study design and geographic factors. However, other factors should be considered. All studies to date have encompassed multiple years to enable analysis of different viral strains as the dominant genotype varies year to year. This inherently introduces a significant confounder with changes between years in staff, clinical practice, herd immunity, etc. In addition, there is increasing evidence of virulence factors encoded in regions of the genome outside the G protein hypervariable region that has been traditionally used for genotyping. Studies in the mouse model have demonstrated that specific sequences within the conserved central domain of the G protein influence RSV binding to the chemokine receptor CX3CR1 impacting host response [61] and sequences contained in the F protein are associated with significant differences in disease severity [62].

The possibility of different RSV genotypes having distinct infective properties is an attractive explanation for the diverse severity of RSV disease which merits further study. It is apparent that the interaction between RSV strain and disease is complex. Whole-genome sequencing perhaps provides the best future opportunity to further our understanding [1].

3. Host factors

3.1 Predisposing health factors

Pre-existing illness and disease have been long recognised as having a significant impact on the severity of RSV disease. RSV infection in children with congenital immunodeficiency (particularly of cell-mediated immunity) is associated with a more severe clinical course [63], and individuals requiring immunosuppressive therapy (such as haemopoietic cell transplant (HCT) recipients and patients undergoing chemotherapy) also experience more sever disease. Following HCT, RSV infection is associated with significant morbidity, including complications such as late graft dysfunction and bronchiolitis obliterans syndrome. Mortality rates range from 7 to 83% depending on a number of risk factors including lymphopenia and high-dose total body irradiation [64–66]. Adult patients with leukaemia are particularly vulnerable to RSV infection with reported mortality rates between 20 and 85% in those developing pneumonia [67] although children with leukaemia appear to follow a more benign clinical course [68].

Pre-existing cardiopulmonary disease has a significant impact on the clinical response to RSV infection. Underlying congenital heart disease in infants and children has long been recognised to be associated with more severe outcomes from RSV, including more frequent hospitalisation, longer lengths of stay and higher rates of intensive care unit admission [69]. Similarly, children with bronchopulmonary disease have markedly increased morbidity and mortality due to RSV [70]. Adults with underlying cardiac and pulmonary diseases are also prone to severe respiratory illnesses with RSV infection [71]. Adults with chronic obstructive pulmonary disease are particularly vulnerable to RSV infection with a high incidence of lower respiratory tract disease and frequent hospitalisation [71].

The impact of RSV at the extremes of age is significant. Premature birth is a significant risk factor for severe RSV disease; those born at less than 32 weeks of gestational age have approximately double the hospitalisation risk of infants born later [72]. Incomplete immunological and pulmonary maturation and reduced transfer of maternal antibodies are all thought to contribute to this increased risk. The burden in the elderly is also significant with evidence that the impact is similar to that of non-pandemic influenza, both in the community and in nursing homes [73]. RSV outbreaks in nursing homes have been well documented, studies reporting infection rates of over 10% with pneumonia in up to 55% of those affected and mortality rates of up to 20% [73]. A recent prospective, international study detected RSV in over 7% of moderate to severe acute respiratory episodes observed in elderly adults living at home and found that the incidence of RSV infection increased with age [13].

3.2 Predisposing airway geometry

The potential impact of reduced premorbid lung function on the response to a subsequent RSV infection has been of interest for many years. Two initial studies published in 1995 demonstrated that a reduced maximum expiratory flow at functional residual capacity (V_{max}FRC—believed to reflect the size of intrapulmonary airways) measured in infancy before any lower respiratory tract illness was associated with subsequent virus-associated wheeze [74, 75]. Subsequently, a large prospective study of 2133 infants who had neonatal lung function performed found that those subsequently hospitalised with RSV infection had significantly decreased lung function compared to those with RSV infection managed in the community [76]. These data together would suggest that congenitally smaller airways may predispose infants to more severe RSV disease.

3.3 Host immune factors

The immune response to infection can be divided into two arms:

1. Innate immunity—this refers to nonspecific defence mechanisms that activate immediately or within hours of exposure to an infecting organism. The efficacy of these mechanisms does not rely on clonal expansion.

2. Adaptive immunity—the adaptive immune response relies on the clonal expansion of antigen-specific lymphocytes and can take several days to complete. A principal feature of the adaptive immune response is the generation of immunological memory enabling a more rapid and effective response to pathogens that have been previously encountered.

3.3.1 Innate immunity

The innate immune response to RSV infection consists of a coordinated response incorporating a variety of cell types and their products. The character of this response is a critical determinant of the outcome of infection. A slow, weak or inappropriate response will result in delayed viral clearance enabling the virus to spread to the lower airway producing enhanced pathology. An inappropriate innate response will also have a direct impact on the nature and efficacy of the adaptive immune response.

The importance of innate immunity is highlighted by genetic association studies which have identified the strongest associations with severe disease due to polymorphisms of the innate immune system at both the allele and genotype level [77, 78].

3.3.1.1 Toll-like receptors

Type I interferons (IFN-I, α/β) are an important part of the innate immune response to viral infection. Various cell intrinsic pattern recognition receptors (PRRs) including the Toll-like receptors (TLR) recognise RSV as foreign and potentially dangerous. This leads to the activation of key transcription factors including interferon regulatory factors which regulate the expression of IFN-I and pro-inflammatory cytokines [79]. IFN-I upregulates transcription of multiple interferon-stimulated genes (ISGs) via the IFN-I receptor, which interfere with viral replication, thus facilitating viral clearance.

TLR polymorphisms have been widely studied for their potential association with severe RSV disease. Tal et al. identified an overrepresentation of a heterozygous genotype in two TLR4 mutations (Asp299Gly and Thr399Ile) among a group of infants necessitating hospitalisation compared to a community-managed group [80]. Similarly, the same mutations were significantly associated with hospitalisation in a group of primarily premature infants with symptomatic RSV infection [81]. However, subsequent studies have failed to confirm these findings [82, 83] although one study has identified significant variability between different RSV epidemics in the genetic risk of severe disease associated with these polymorphisms [83]. This highlights the complex interplay between host genetic factors and the predominant circulating viral strain.

3.3.1.2 Surfactant proteins

The surfactant proteins (SPs) primarily reduce surface tension of the alveoli to prevent lung collapse but also make a significant contribution to innate immunity. In vitro, SP-A enhances uptake of RSV by macrophages, reduces RSV-induced suppression of host cell tumour necrosis factor-α (TNF-α) and augments the production of anti-inflammatory interleukin-10 (IL-10) [84]. SP-D-deficient mice develop severe disease on exposure to RSV and have delayed viral clearance [85]. Studies on ventilated infants with RSV infection have demonstrated low surfactant activity and reduced levels of SP-A, SP-B and SP-D compared to controls [86, 87]. In addition, genetic analyses have identified certain polymorphisms of the surfactant proteins that are associated with severe disease in RSV-infected infants [88, 89].

3.3.1.3 Inflammatory mediators

The initial contact between RSV and the host is typically at the nasal epithelium. The epithelial surfaces form a physical barrier that is impermeable to most infectious agents, acting as the first line of defence against invading organisms. In response to contact with RSV, the epithelium also releases a variety of pro-inflammatory mediators and cytokines that play an important part in the innate immune response. A number of in vitro studies have demonstrated the production of IL-1; IL-6; IL-8; tumour necrosis factor-α; regulated upon activation, normal T-cell expressed and presumably secreted (RANTES); and CXCL8 by RSV-infected primary airway epithelial cell cultures [90–92]. Macrophages and neutrophils are important phagocytes but also produce a wide range of immunological mediators, including MIP-1α, RANTES, IL-1, IL-6 and IL-8, when infected with RSV in vitro [93, 94]. Such mediators have a significant impact on both early inflammation as well as subsequent immunological responses. For example, IL-8 is chemotactic for neutrophils as well as being a potent activator. Similarly, MIP-1α and RANTES activate both monocytes and eosinophils as well as being potent $CD4^+$ T-cell chemoattractants.

Respiratory secretions from infants and children infected with RSV have been found to contain many of these mediators [38, 95–97]. Some studies have also identified correlates between certain inflammatory mediator concentrations and disease severity. Higher levels of IL-8 have been identified in severe disease with a strong correlation with oxygen requirement and need for ventilation [96, 98]. Nasal concentrations of MIP-1α are significantly increased in children with RSV bronchiolitis that require oxygen therapy [99] and in RSV-infected adults that require hospitalisation [100].

There has been much interest in the contribution of RANTES, a potent chemoattractant for eosinophils, T cells and monocytes, to the pathogenesis of RSV disease. RANTES levels in tracheal aspirates have been found to correlate inversely with markers of disease severity in RSV bronchiolitis [95], and the ratio of TNF-receptor to RANTES in nasopharyngeal aspirates is significantly raised in infants with severe RSV disease [101]. The potential protective impact of RANTES has been further explored through analysis of promoter and intronic polymorphisms in the RANTES gene. Certain polymorphisms (e.g., −403 G/A) have been associated with reduced disease severity and greater production of RANTES [102, 103].

3.3.1.4 Eosinophils

Eosinophils have been traditionally regarded as important in the innate immune response to helminthic infection although several studies have suggested their possible contribution to RSV immunity. Eosinophil cationic protein (ECP), a cytotoxic protein released with eosinophil activation, is found in nasal lavage fluid and serum from children with severe RSV infection [104]. ECP levels in nasopharyngeal secretions have been found to correlate with disease severity [105, 106] suggesting a role for the eosinophil in the pathogenesis of RSV disease.

3.3.2 Adaptive immunity

3.3.2.1 Humoral immunity

The developing foetus acquires maternal IgG antibodies to RSV through the placenta actively. The transfer rate gradually increases from 30 weeks of gestation to a maximum between 38 and 40 weeks. Following birth, levels of neutralising antibody slowly diminish with a mean half-life of 26 days [107]. The quantity of antibody transferred is important in protecting infants against infection; higher specific antibody titres are associated with milder disease following RSV infection [108]. Infants also acquire antibodies from the mother through breast feeding with breast fed infants having significantly reduced oxygen requirement and length of stay following hospitalisation with RSV bronchiolitis [109].

There is considerable variability in the humoral response of infants to primary infection. During the first year of life, there is rapid maturation of the immune system, and this may account for much of this variability. In the first 6 months of life, the serum IgA response is greater than that of IgG [110]. In older children, there is a predominant rise in IgG levels with IgG1 and IgG3 subclasses accounting for the major part of this response [110], whereas IgG1 and IgG2 subclasses form the bulk of the adult response [111]. As well as these qualitative differences in antibody response with age, there is also quantitative variation with generally very low titres of antibody produced in early infancy. The antibody titres against both the F and G surface proteins of RSV in infancy are 10 to 12 times lower than those observed in children over 12 months of age [112]. This blunted response appears to be caused by a combination of factors including the presence of residual maternal antibody and immaturity of the immune system [113].

Murine studies have demonstrated that the humoral response is an important factor in RSV disease severity. B-cell-depleted mice, which consequently have no antibody response to infection, experience greater illness on primary RSV infection [114]. Similarly, higher neutralising antibody titres in children are associated with a lower incidence of severe lower respiratory tract disease once infected with RSV. Clinical severity scores inversely correlate with antibody titres to the F protein in infants with RSV infection [115], and therapeutic trials of polyclonal and monoclonal antibodies have demonstrated reduced disease severity in treated infants [116, 117].

3.3.2.2 Cell-mediated immunity

The cellular arm of the adaptive immune response is orchestrated primarily by cytotoxic T lymphocytes (CTLs) and T-helper (Th) lymphocytes. Cell-mediated immunity is extremely important for the eradication and abrogation of the clinical response to RSV infection as highlighted by the severe impact of infection in individuals with severe congenital/acquired impairment of cellular immunity [63, 118].

3.3.2.2.1 Cytotoxic T lymphocytes (CD8⁺ T cells)

CTLs are pivotal for the control of many intracellular pathogens and have the capacity to differentiate into long-lived memory CTLs which provide a rapid, robust response to subsequent infection. CTLs have been found to have an important role in clearing RSV during animal studies. Mice that have been rendered athymic are unable to produce a CTL response to RSV infection and become chronically infected. Clearance of the virus can be subsequently achieved by injecting the mice with primed RSV-specific CTLs [119]. There is also some evidence that CTLs can contribute to severe disease if produced in large numbers [120].

Unfortunately, the role of CTLs in human RSV infection has been little studied largely due to the relatively modest RSV-specific T-cell responses observed in the blood and the low numbers of RSV-specific T-cell memory cells present between infections. Using HLA tetrameric staining, RSV-specific $CD8^+$ T cells were analysed in bronchoalveolar lavage fluid and blood specimens from infants requiring ventilatory support for RSV bronchiolitis. RSV-specific T-cell numbers peaked in blood around days 9–12 (at the time of recovery), and there was no correlation between cell numbers and parameters of disease severity [121]. A similar pattern is observed in experimental infection of adult volunteers where antigen-specific $CD8^+$ T-cell numbers peak 10 days after initial infection at approximately the same time as a fall in viral load and resolution of symptoms [122]. This would perhaps suggest an important contribution to viral clearance although the impact of CTLs on disease severity in man remains undefined.

3.3.2.2.2 T-helper lymphocytes ($CD4^+$ T cells)

$CD4^+$ T cells recognise antigens presented on MHC class II molecules, which are found on antigen-presenting cells. They respond by releasing cytokines which play a major role in instigating and shaping adaptive immune responses. The cytokines produced have been used to differentiate these cells into the two major classes of effector T cell—T helper (Th) 1 (producing type 1 cytokines) and Th2 (producing type 2 cytokines) [123]. In general, type 1 cytokines (such as interferon-gamma (IFN-γ) and IL-12) favour the development of a strong cellular immune response and are an important component of an effective response to intracellular pathogens including viruses. Type 2 cytokines (such as IL-4 and IL-5) favour a strong humoral response to infection by promoting B-cell proliferation and increased production of antibodies. Type 2 cytokines also mediate allergic responses. Cross regulation occurs between the two responses, and responses deviated toward type 2 or away from type 1 are associated with more severe disease in several infectious disease model [124, 125].

Indirect evidence suggests that T-helper lymphocytes have a significant role in RSV disease with $CD4^+$ T cells constituting the largest lymphocyte population in bronchoalveolar lavage fluid obtained from infants ventilated for RSV bronchiolitis [126]. Subsequent studies have focussed on the exact nature of this $CD4^+$ T-cell response.

Murine studies have demonstrated that prior sensitisation to RSV surface proteins followed 3 weeks later by RSV infection can induce polarised cytokine responses which follow broad type 1 and type 2 repertoires [127]. Type 2 responses were associated with enhanced disease characterised by pulmonary haemorrhage and eosinophilia while those with type 1 responses had reduced immunopathology and enhanced viral clearance [128]. A type 2 cytokine response also correlates with quantitated pulmonary pathology following primary RSV infection of BALB/c mice [129].

Multiple human studies have examined type 1 and type 2 immune responses to RSV and have largely identified a similar predominance of type 2 cytokines in those with more severe disease. Type 1 cytokines (including IFN-γ and TNF-α) are increased in the circulation, the nose and lung during an RSV LRTI [96, 130, 131]. Lower IFN-γ levels are associated with increased severity scores, hypoxia and need for ventilation [97, 131–134]. Type 2 cytokines (including IL-4, IL-10 and IL-13) are also increased in the blood, nose and lung during RSV LRTI [95, 132, 135]. However, higher type 2 cytokine levels are generally associated with more severe disease. Systemic IL-10 levels correlate with disease severity in RSV LRTI [136, 137] although respiratory tract IL-10 levels would appear to be associated with milder disease features [95].

Multiple studies have also evaluated the type 1/type 2 immune balance through the quantification of cytokine ratio. The ratio of IL-4 to IFN-γ is raised both systemically and in the respiratory tract in patients with bronchiolitis that require oxygen therapy suggesting a skew towards type 2 responses [138, 139]. Similarly, IL-4:IFN-γ and IL-10:IL-12 ratios are raised in nasal lavage obtained from infants with RSV who develop bronchiolitis compared to those that develop signs of an URTI only [23], and type 2 cytokines predominate in nasopharyngeal specimens from children with hypoxic RSV LRTI [96].

Overall, current evidence would support a bias towards a type 2 T-helper cell response in severe RSV infection. Further studies are, however, required to confirm these findings and would ideally analyse prospectively the cytokine response both systemically and within the airway. Such studies should, also, examine both children and adults with RSV infection using relevant study groups (URTI, LRTI) and strictly control for potential confounding factors such as sampling times (relative to infection onset) and age differences between groups.

3.3.2.2.3 Regulatory T cells

Regulatory T cells (Tregs) are immunoregulating cells that maintain the immunological equilibrium by controlling effector T-cell activation and hence preventing tissue damage during the immune response to infections [140]. Animal studies in Treg-depleted mice have highlighted their importance. RSV infection of Treg-depleted mice results in severe disease with a significantly elevated viral load and an exuberant cytotoxic T-cell response highlighting the importance of Tregs for both viral clearance and control of the RSV-specific T-cell response [141]. A recent study of infants with severe bronchiolitis demonstrated a prolonged reduction in Tregs in these patients compared to a similarly aged, healthy control group [142]. While intriguing, further studies are required to confirm this finding and to clarify the role of Tregs in severity of RSV disease.

4. Conclusion

The broad spectrum of disease due to RSV infection likely represents a complex interplay between multiple viral and host factors. Despite significant research in this area, our understanding of the relative importance of each factor is limited although recent studies that have examined multiple components of the virus-host interaction have provided some insight. Individual viral strains have differing infective properties which primarily determine RSV virulence alongside other factors such as viral load. The host immune response is increasingly recognised as an important determinant of disease severity. Other host factors including underlying immunological/cardiopulmonary disease and small airway geometry in infancy also appear to have an important impact.

Each year 2–3% of all infants require hospitalisation due to RSV outbreaks [6]. These epidemics result in substantial healthcare costs with direct medical costs for children <5 years old amounting to over $600 million in the United States alone [143]. Despite the substantial impact of RSV, advances in effective prevention and treatment have been slow. Future studies that consider fully the contribution of both viral and host factors in the pathogenesis of severe disease will undoubtedly facilitate the development of effective therapies.

Conflicts of interest

Dr. Legg has no potential conflicts of interest.

Author details

Julian P. Legg[1,2,3]

1 Department of Paediatric Respiratory Medicine, Southampton Children's Hospital, Southampton, UK

2 Southampton NIHR Respiratory Biomedical Research Unit, Southampton General Hospital, Southampton, UK

3 Clinical and Experimental Sciences, University of Southampton Faculty of Medicine, Southampton General Hospital, Southampton, UK

*Address all correspondence to: jpl2@soton.ac.uk

References

[1] Griffiths C, Drews SJ, Marchant DJ. Respiratory syncytial virus: Infection, detection, and new options for prevention and treatment. Clinical Microbiology Reviews. 2017;**30**:277-319. DOI: 10.1128/CMR.00010-16

[2] Borchers AT, Chang C, Gershwin ME, Gershwin LJ. Respiratory syncytial virus—A comprehensive review. Clinical Reviews in Allergy and Immunology. 2013;**45**:331-379. DOI: 10.1007/s12016-013-8368-9

[3] Glezen WP, Taber LH, Frank AL, Kasel JA. Risk of primary infection and reinfection with respiratory syncytial virus. American Journal of Diseases of Children (1960). 1986;**140**:543-546

[4] Sims DG, Downham MA, McQuillin J, Gardner PS. Respiratory syncytial virus infection in North-East England. British Medical Journal. 1976;**2**:1095-1098. DOI: 10.1136/bmj.2.6044.1095

[5] Fields BN, Knipe DM, Howley PM. Fields Virology. Philadelphia: Wolters Kluwer Health/Lippincott Williams & Wilkins; 2013

[6] Hall CB, Weinberg GA, Iwane MK, Blumkin AK, Edwards KM, Staat MA, et al. The burden of respiratory syncytial virus infection in young children. The New England Journal of Medicine. 2009;**360**:588-598. DOI: 10.1056/NEJMoa0804877

[7] Nair H, Nokes DJ, Gessner BD, Dherani M, Madhi SA, Singleton RJ, et al. Global burden of acute lower respiratory infections due to respiratory syncytial virus in young children: A systematic review and meta-analysis. The Lancet. 2010;**375**:1545-1555. DOI: 10.1016/S0140-6736(10)60206-1

[8] Lozano R, Naghavi M, Foreman K, Lim S, Shibuya K, Aboyans V, et al. Global and regional mortality from 235 causes of death for 20 age groups in 1990 and 2010: A systematic analysis for the global burden of disease study 2010. Lancet (Lond, Engl). 2012;**380**:2095-2128. DOI: 10.1016/S0140-6736(12)61728-0

[9] Hall CB, Geiman JM, Biggar R, Kotok DI, Hogan PM, Douglas GR. Respiratory syncytial virus infections within families. The New England Journal of Medicine. 1976;**294**:414-419. DOI: 10.1056/NEJM197602192940803

[10] Hall WJ, Hall CB, Speers DM. Respiratory syncytial virus infection in adults: Clinical, virologic, and serial pulmonary function studies. Annals of Internal Medicine. 1978;**88**:203-205

[11] Hall CB, Walsh EE, Long CE, Schnabel KC. Immunity to and frequency of reinfection with respiratory syncytial virus. The Journal of Infectious Diseases. 1991;**163**:693-698. DOI: 10.1093/infdis/163.4.693

[12] Dowell SF, Anderson LJ, Gary HE, Erdman DD, Plouffe JF, File TM, et al. Respiratory syncytial virus is an important cause of community-acquired lower respiratory infection among hospitalized adults. The Journal of Infectious Diseases. 1996;**174**:456-462. DOI: 10.1093/infdis/174.3.456

[13] Falsey AR, McElhaney JE, Beran J, van Essen GA, Duval X, Esen M, et al. Respiratory syncytial virus and other respiratory viral infections in older adults with moderate to severe influenza-like illness. The Journal of Infectious Diseases. 2014;**209**:1873-1881. DOI: 10.1093/infdis/jit839

[14] Morris JA, Saglam M, Bozeman FM. Recovery of a new syncytium virus from a cottontail rabbit. The Journal of Infectious Diseases. 1965;**115**:495-499

[15] Chanock R, Finberg L. Recovery from infants with respiratory illness of a virus related to chimpanzee coryza agent (CCA). II. Epidemiologic aspects of infection in infants and young children. American Journal of Hygiene. 1957;**66**:291-300

[16] Mcclelland L, Hilleman MR, Hamparian VV, Ketler A, Reilly CM, Cornfeld D, et al. Studies of acute respiratory illnesses caused by respiratory syncytial virus. 2. Epidemiology and assessment of importance. The New England Journal of Medicine. 1961;**264**:1169-1175. DOI: 10.1056/NEJM196106082642301

[17] Weiland O, Braconier JH, Frydén A, Norkrans G, Reichard O, Uhnoo I. Influence of pre-treatment factors on outcome of interferon-alpha treatment of patients with chronic hepatitis C. Scandinavian Journal of Infectious Diseases. 1999;**31**:115-118

[18] Mellors JW. Plasma viral load and $CD4^+$ lymphocytes as prognostic markers of HIV-1 infection. Annals of Internal Medicine. 1997;**126**:946. DOI: 10.7326/0003-4819-126-12-199706150-00003

[19] DeVincenzo JP, El Saleeby CM, Bush AJ. Respiratory syncytial virus load predicts disease severity in previously healthy infants. The Journal of Infectious Diseases. 2005;**191**:1861-1868. DOI: 10.1086/430008

[20] Houben ML, Coenjaerts FEJ, Rossen JWA, Belderbos ME, Hofland RW, Kimpen JLL, et al. Disease severity and viral load are correlated in infants with primary respiratory syncytial virus infection in the community. Journal of Medical Virology. 2010;**82**:1266-1271. DOI: 10.1002/jmv.21771

[21] Fodha I, Vabret A, Ghedira L, Seboui H, Chouchane S, Dewar J, et al. Respiratory syncytial virus infections in hospitalized infants: Association between viral load, virus subgroup, and disease severity. Journal of Medical Virology. 2007;**79**:1951-1958. DOI: 10.1002/jmv.21026

[22] de Souza APD, Leitão LA de A, Luisi F, Souza RG, Coutinho SE, da Silva JR, et al. Lack of association between viral load and severity of acute bronchiolitis in infants. Jornal Brasileiro de Pneumologia. 2016;**42**:261-265. DOI: 10.1590/S1806-37562015000000241

[23] Legg JP, Hussain IR, Warner JA, Johnston SL, Warner JO. Type 1 and type 2 cytokine imbalance in acute respiratory syncytial virus bronchiolitis. American Journal of Respiratory and Critical Care Medicine. 2003;**168**:633-639. DOI: 10.1164/rccm.200210-1148OC

[24] Martin ET, Kuypers J, Heugel J, Englund JA. Clinical disease and viral load in children infected with respiratory syncytial virus or human metapneumovirus. Diagnostic Microbiology and Infectious Disease. 2008;**62**:382-388. DOI: 10.1016/j.diagmicrobio.2008.08.002

[25] Garcia-Mauriño C, Moore-Clingenpeel M, Thomas J, Mertz S, Cohen DM, Ramilo O, et al. Viral load dynamics and clinical disease severity in infants with respiratory syncytial virus infection. The Journal of Infectious Diseases. 2019;**219**:1207-1215. DOI: 10.1093/infdis/jiy655

[26] Thwaites RS, Coates M, Ito K, Ghazaly M, Feather C, Abdulla F, et al. Reduced nasal viral load and IFN responses in infants with respiratory syncytial virus bronchiolitis and respiratory failure. American Journal of Respiratory and Critical Care Medicine. 2018;**198**:1074-1084. DOI: 10.1164/rccm.201712-2567OC

[27] El Saleeby CM, Bush AJ, Harrison LM, Aitken JA, DeVincenzo JP.

Respiratory syncytial virus load, viral dynamics, and disease severity in previously healthy naturally infected children. The Journal of Infectious Diseases. 2011;**204**:996-1002. DOI: 10.1093/infdis/jir494

[28] Anderson LJ, Hierholzer JC, Tsou C, Hendry RM, Fernie BF, Stone Y, et al. Antigenic characterization of respiratory syncytial virus strains with monoclonal antibodies. The Journal of Infectious Diseases. 1985;**151**:626-633. DOI: 10.1093/infdis/151.4.626

[29] Peret TC, Hall CB, Hammond GW, Piedra PA, Storch GA, Sullender WM, et al. Circulation patterns of group A and B human respiratory syncytial virus genotypes in 5 communities in North America. The Journal of Infectious Diseases. 2000;**181**:1891-1896. DOI: 10.1086/315508

[30] Hendry RM, Talis AL, Godfrey E, Anderson LJ, Fernie BF, McIntosh K. Concurrent circulation of antigenically distinct strains of respiratory syncytial virus during community outbreaks. The Journal of Infectious Diseases. 1986;**153**:291-297. DOI: 10.1093/infdis/153.2.291

[31] Hall CB, Walsh EE, Schnabel KC, Long CE, McConnochie KM, Hildreth SW, et al. Occurrence of groups a and B of respiratory syncytial virus over 15 years: Associated epidemiologic and clinical characteristics in hospitalized and ambulatory children. The Journal of Infectious Diseases. 1990;**162**:1283-1290. DOI: 10.1093/infdis/162.6.1283

[32] Jafri HS, Wu X, Makari D, Henrickson KJ. Distribution of respiratory syncytial virus subtypes A and B among infants presenting to the emergency department with lower respiratory tract infection or apnea. The Pediatric Infectious Disease Journal. 2013;**32**:335-340. DOI: 10.1097/INF.0b013e318282603a

[33] Tabarani CM, Bonville CA, Suryadevara M, Branigan P, Wang D, Huang D, et al. Novel inflammatory markers, clinical risk factors and virus type associated with severe respiratory syncytial virus infection. The Pediatric Infectious Disease Journal. 2013;**32**:e437-e442. DOI: 10.1097/INF.0b013e3182a14407

[34] Rodriguez-Fernandez R, Tapia LI, Yang C-F, Torres JP, Chavez-Bueno S, Garcia C, et al. Respiratory syncytial virus genotypes, host immune profiles, and disease severity in young children hospitalized with bronchiolitis. The Journal of Infectious Diseases. 2018;**217**:24-34. DOI: 10.1093/infdis/jix543

[35] Laham FR, Mansbach JM, Piedra PA, Hasegawa K, Sullivan AF, Espinola JA, et al. Clinical profiles of respiratory syncytial virus subtypes a AND B among children hospitalized with bronchiolitis. The Pediatric Infectious Disease Journal. 2017;**36**:808-810. DOI: 10.1097/INF.0000000000001596

[36] Comas-García A, Noyola DE, Cadena-Mota S, Rico-Hernández M, Bernal-Silva S. Respiratory syncytial virus-a ON1 genotype emergence in Central Mexico in 2009 and evidence of multiple duplication events. The Journal of Infectious Diseases. 2018;**217**:1089-1098. DOI: 10.1093/infdis/jiy025

[37] McIntosh ED, De Silva LM, Oates RK. Clinical severity of respiratory syncytial virus group A and B infection in Sydney, Australia. The Pediatric Infectious Disease Journal. 1993;**12**:815-819

[38] Hornsleth A, Klug B, Nir M, Johansen J, Hansen KS, Christensen LS, et al. Severity of respiratory syncytial virus disease related to type and genotype of virus and to cytokine values in nasopharyngeal secretions. The

Pediatric Infectious Disease Journal. 1998;**17**:1114-1121

[39] Panayiotou C, Richter J, Koliou M, Kalogirou N, Georgiou E, Christodoulou C. Epidemiology of respiratory syncytial virus in children in Cyprus during three consecutive winter seasons (2010-2013): Age distribution, seasonality and association between prevalent genotypes and disease severity. Epidemiology and Infection. 2014;**142**:2406-2411. DOI: 10.1017/S0950268814000028

[40] Melero JA, García-Barreno B, Martínez I, Pringle CR, Cane PA. Antigenic structure, evolution and immunobiology of human respiratory syncytial virus attachment (G) protein. The Journal of General Virology. 1997;**78**(Pt 10):2411-2418. DOI: 10.1099/0022-1317-78-10-2411

[41] Scholtissek C. Molecular evolution of influenza viruses. Virus Genes. 1995;**11**:209-215

[42] Cane PA, Pringle CR. Molecular epidemiology of respiratory syncytial virus: A review of the use of reverse transcription-polymerase chain reaction in the analysis of genetic variability. Electrophoresis. 1995;**16**:329-333

[43] Sullender WM. Respiratory syncytial virus genetic and antigenic diversity. Clinical Microbiology Reviews. 2000;**13**:1-15. Table of contents. DOI: 10.1128/cmr.13.1.1-15.2000

[44] Coggins WB, Lefkowitz EJ, Sullender WM. Genetic variability among group A and group B respiratory syncytial viruses in a children's hospital. Journal of Clinical Microbiology. 1998;**36**:3552-3557

[45] Song J, Wang H, Shi J, Cui A, Huang Y, Sun L, et al. Emergence of BA9 genotype of human respiratory syncytial virus subgroup B in China from 2006 to 2014. Scientific Reports. 2017;7:16765. DOI: 10.1038/s41598-017-17055-0

[46] Cane PA. Molecular epidemiology of respiratory syncytial virus. Reviews in Medical Virology. 2001;**11**:103-116. DOI: 10.1002/rmv.305

[47] Agoti CN, Mwihuri AG, Sande CJ, Onyango CO, Medley GF, Cane PA, et al. Genetic relatedness of infecting and reinfecting respiratory syncytial virus strains identified in a birth cohort from rural Kenya. The Journal of Infectious Diseases. 2012;**206**:1532-1541. DOI: 10.1093/infdis/jis570

[48] Botosso VF, Zanotto PM de A, Ueda M, Arruda E, Gilio AE, Vieira SE, et al. Positive selection results in frequent reversible amino acid replacements in the G protein gene of human respiratory syncytial virus. PLoS Pathogens. 2009;**5**:e1000254. DOI: 10.1371/journal.ppat.1000254

[49] Tan L, Lemey P, Houspie L, Viveen MC, Jansen NJG, van LAM, et al. Genetic variability among complete human respiratory syncytial virus subgroup a genomes: Bridging molecular evolutionary dynamics and epidemiology. PLoS One. 2012;7:e51439. DOI: 10.1371/journal.pone.0051439

[50] Trento A, Galiano M, Videla C, Carballal G, García-Barreno B, Melero JA, et al. Major changes in the G protein of human respiratory syncytial virus isolates introduced by a duplication of 60 nucleotides. The Journal of General Virology. 2003;**84**:3115-3120. DOI: 10.1099/vir.0.19357-0

[51] Trento A, Casas I, Calderón A, Garcia-Garcia ML, Calvo C, Perez-Breña P, et al. Ten years of global evolution of the human respiratory syncytial virus BA genotype with a 60-nucleotide duplication in the G protein gene. Journal of Virology.

2010;**84**:7500-7512. DOI: 10.1128/JVI.00345-10

[52] Houspie L, Lemey P, Keyaerts E, Reijmen E, Vergote V, Vankeerberghen A, et al. Circulation of HRSV in Belgium: From multiple genotype circulation to prolonged circulation of predominant genotypes. PLoS One. 2013;**8**:e60416. DOI: 10.1371/journal.pone.0060416

[53] van Niekerk S, Venter M. Replacement of previously circulating respiratory syncytial virus subtype B strains with the BA genotype in South Africa. Journal of Virology. 2011;**85**:8789-8797. DOI: 10.1128/JVI.02623-10

[54] Eshaghi A, Duvvuri VR, Lai R, Nadarajah JT, Li A, Patel SN, et al. Genetic variability of human respiratory syncytial virus a strains circulating in Ontario: A novel genotype with a 72 nucleotide G gene duplication. PLoS One. 2012;7:e32807. DOI: 10.1371/journal.pone.0032807

[55] Gaymard A, Bouscambert-Duchamp M, Pichon M, Frobert E, Vallee J, Lina B, et al. Genetic characterization of respiratory syncytial virus highlights a new BA genotype and emergence of the ON1 genotype in Lyon, France, between 2010 and 2014. Journal of Clinical Virology: The Official Publication of the Pan American Society for Clinical Virology. 2018;**102**:12-18. DOI: 10.1016/j.jcv.2018.02.004

[56] Hirano E, Kobayashi M, Tsukagoshi H, Yoshida LM, Kuroda M, Noda M, et al. Molecular evolution of human respiratory syncytial virus attachment glycoprotein (G) gene of new genotype ON1 and ancestor NA1. Infection, Genetics and Evolution: Journal of Molecular Epidemiology and Evolutionary Genetics of Infectious Diseases. 2014;**28**:183-191. DOI: 10.1016/j.meegid.2014.09.030

[57] Midulla F, Nenna R, Scagnolari C, Petrarca L, Frassanito A, Viscido A, et al. How respiratory syncytial virus genotypes influence the clinical course in infants hospitalized for bronchiolitis. The Journal of Infectious Diseases. 2019;**219**:526-534. DOI: 10.1093/infdis/jiy496

[58] Esposito S, Piralla A, Zampiero A, Bianchini S, Di Pietro G, Scala A, et al. Characteristics and their clinical relevance of respiratory syncytial virus types and genotypes circulating in northern Italy in five consecutive winter seasons. PLoS One. 2015;**10**:e0129369. DOI: 10.1371/journal.pone.0129369

[59] Tabatabai J, Prifert C, Pfeil J, Grulich-Henn J, Schnitzler P. Novel respiratory syncytial virus (RSV) genotype ON1 predominates in Germany during winter season 2012-13. PLoS One. 2014;**9**:e109191. DOI: 10.1371/journal.pone.0109191

[60] Yoshihara K, Le MN, Okamoto M, Wadagni ACA, Nguyen HA, Toizumi M, et al. Association of RSV-A ON1 genotype with increased pediatric acute lower respiratory tract infection in Vietnam. Scientific Reports. 2016;**6**. DOI: 10.1038/srep27856

[61] Boyoglu-Barnum S, Todd SO, Meng J, Barnum TR, Chirkova T, Haynes LM, et al. Mutating the CX3C motif in the G protein should make a live respiratory syncytial virus vaccine safer and more effective. Journal of Virology. 2017;**91**:e02059-e02016. DOI: 10.1128/JVI.02059-16

[62] Currier MG, Lee S, Stobart CC, Hotard AL, Villenave R, Meng J, et al. EGFR interacts with the fusion protein of respiratory syncytial virus strain 2-20 and mediates infection and mucin expression. PLoS Pathogens. 2016;**12**. DOI: 10.1371/journal.ppat.1005622

[63] Hall CB, Powell KR, MacDonald NE, Gala CL, Menegus ME, Suffin SC, et al. Respiratory syncytial viral infection in children with

compromised immune function. The New England Journal of Medicine. 1986;**315**:77-81. DOI: 10.1056/NEJM198607103150201

[64] Erard V, Chien JW, Kim HW, Nichols WG, Flowers ME, Martin PJ, et al. Airflow decline after myeloablative allogeneic hematopoietic cell transplantation: The role of community respiratory viruses. The Journal of Infectious Diseases. 2006;**193**:1619-1625. DOI: 10.1086/504268

[65] Avetisyan G, Mattsson J, Sparrelid E, Ljungman P. Respiratory syncytial virus infection in recipients of allogeneic stem-cell transplantation: A retrospective study of the incidence, clinical features, and outcome. Transplantation. 2009;**88**:1222-1226. DOI: 10.1097/TP.0b013e3181bb477e

[66] Khanna N, Widmer AF, Decker M, Steffen I, Halter J, Heim D, et al. Respiratory syncytial virus infection in patients with hematological diseases: Single-center study and review of the literature. Clinical Infectious Diseases: An Official Publication of the Infectious Diseases Society of America. 2008;**46**:402-412. DOI: 10.1086/525263

[67] Torres HA, Aguilera EA, Mattiuzzi GN, Cabanillas ME, Rohatgi N, Sepulveda CA, et al. Characteristics and outcome of respiratory syncytial virus infection in patients with leukemia. Haematologica. 2007;**92**:1216-1223

[68] Torres JP, De la Maza V, Kors L, Villarroel M, Piemonte P, Izquierdo G, et al. Respiratory viral infections and coinfections in children with cancer, fever and neutropenia: Clinical outcome of infections caused by different respiratory viruses. The Pediatric Infectious Disease Journal. 2016;**35**:949-954. DOI: 10.1097/INF.0000000000001209

[69] Checchia PA, Paes B, Bont L, Manzoni P, Simões EAF, Fauroux B, et al. Defining the risk and associated morbidity and mortality of severe respiratory syncytial virus infection among infants with congenital heart disease. Infectious Disease and Therapy. 2017;**6**:37-56. DOI: 10.1007/s40121-016-0142-x

[70] Paes B, Fauroux B, Figueras-Aloy J, Bont L, Checchia PA, Simões EAF, et al. Defining the risk and associated morbidity and mortality of severe respiratory syncytial virus infection among infants with chronic lung disease. Infectious Disease and Therapy. 2016;**5**:453-471. DOI: 10.1007/s40121-016-0137-7

[71] Falsey AR, Hennessey PA, Formica MA, Cox C, Walsh EE. Respiratory syncytial virus infection in elderly and high-risk adults. The New England Journal of Medicine. 2005;**352**:1749-1759. DOI: 10.1056/NEJMoa043951

[72] Langley GFM, Anderson LJ. Epidemiology and prevention of respiratory syncytial virus infections among infants and Young children [review]. ET Journal. 2011;**30**:510-517. DOI: 10.1097/INF.0b013e3182184ae7

[73] Haber N. Respiratory syncytial virus infection in elderly adults. Médecine et Maladies Infectieuses. 2018;**48**:377-382. DOI: 10.1016/j.medmal.2018.01.008

[74] Martinez FD, Wright AL, Taussig LM, Holberg CJ, Halonen M, Morgan WJ. Asthma and wheezing in the first six years of life. The Group Health Medical Associates. The New England Journal of Medicine. 1995;**332**:133-138. DOI: 10.1056/NEJM199501193320301

[75] Young S, O'Keeffe PT, Arnott J, Landau LI. Lung function, airway responsiveness, and respiratory symptoms before and after bronchiolitis. Archives of Disease in

Childhood. 1995;**72**:16-24. DOI: 10.1136/adc.72.1.16

[76] Zomer-Kooijker K, Uiterwaal CSPM, van der GAC, Wilbrink B, Bont LJ, van der ECK. Decreased lung function precedes severe respiratory syncytial virus infection and post-respiratory syncytial virus wheeze in term infants. The European Respiratory Journal. 2014;**44**:666-674. DOI: 10.1183/09031936.00009314

[77] Janssen R, Bont L, Siezen CLE, Hodemaekers HM, Ermers MJ, Doornbos G, et al. Genetic susceptibility to respiratory syncytial virus bronchiolitis is predominantly associated with innate immune genes. The Journal of Infectious Diseases. 2007;**196**:826-834. DOI: 10.1086/520886

[78] Siezen CLE, Bont L, Hodemaekers HM, Ermers MJ, Doornbos G, Van't Slot R, et al. Genetic susceptibility to respiratory syncytial virus bronchiolitis in preterm children is associated with airway remodeling genes and innate immune genes. The Pediatric Infectious Disease Journal. 2009;**28**:333-335. DOI: 10.1097/INF.0b013e31818e2aa9

[79] Chan YK, Gack MU. Viral evasion of intracellular DNA and RNA sensing. Nature Reviews. Microbiology. 2016;**14**:360-373. DOI: 10.1038/nrmicro.2016.45

[80] Tal G, Mandelberg A, Dalal I, Cesar K, Somekh E, Tal A, et al. Association between common Toll-like receptor 4 mutations and severe respiratory syncytial virus disease. The Journal of Infectious Diseases. 2004;**189**:2057-2063. DOI: 10.1086/420830

[81] Awomoyi AA, Rallabhandi P, Pollin TI, Lorenz E, Sztein MB, Boukhvalova MS, et al. Association of TLR4 polymorphisms with symptomatic respiratory syncytial virus infection in high-risk infants and young children. Journal of Immunology (Baltimore, MD) (1950). 2007;**179**:3171-3177. DOI: 10.4049/jimmunol.179.5.3171

[82] Paulus SC, Hirschfeld AF, Victor RE, Brunstein J, Thomas E, Turvey SE. Common human Toll-like receptor 4 polymorphisms--role in susceptibility to respiratory syncytial virus infection and functional immunological relevance. Clinical Immunology (Orlando, FL). 2007;**123**:252-257. DOI: 10.1016/j.clim.2007.03.003

[83] Löfgren J, Marttila R, Renko M, Rämet M, Hallman M. Toll-like receptor 4 Asp299Gly polymorphism in respiratory syncytial virus epidemics. Pediatric Pulmonology. 2010;**45**:687-692. DOI: 10.1002/ppul.21248

[84] Barr FE, Pedigo H, Johnson TR, Shepherd VL. Surfactant protein-a enhances uptake of respiratory syncytial virus by monocytes and U937 macrophages. American Journal of Respiratory Cell and Molecular Biology. 2000;**23**:586-592. DOI: 10.1165/ajrcmb.23.5.3771

[85] LeVine AM, Elliott J, Whitsett JA, Srikiatkhachorn A, Crouch E, DeSilva N, et al. Surfactant protein-d enhances phagocytosis and pulmonary clearance of respiratory syncytial virus. American Journal of Respiratory Cell and Molecular Biology. 2004;**31**:193-199. DOI: 10.1165/rcmb.2003-0107OC

[86] Skelton R, Holland P, Darowski M, Chetcuti PA, Morgan LW, Harwood JL. Abnormal surfactant composition and activity in severe bronchiolitis. Acta Paediatrica (Oslo, Norway: 1992). 1999;**88**:942-946

[87] Kerr MH, Paton JY. Surfactant protein levels in severe respiratory syncytial virus infection. American Journal of Respiratory and Critical Care

Medicine. 1999;**159**:1115-1118. DOI: 10.1164/ajrccm.159.4.9709065

[88] Lahti M, Löfgren J, Marttila R, Renko M, Klaavuniemi T, Haataja R, et al. Surfactant protein D gene polymorphism associated with severe respiratory syncytial virus infection. Pediatric Research. 2002;**51**:696. DOI: 10.1203/00006450-200206000-00006

[89] Saleeby CME, Li R, Somes GW, Dahmer MK, Quasney MW, DeVincenzo JP. Surfactant protein A2 polymorphisms and disease severity in a respiratory syncytial virus-infected population. The Journal of Pediatrics. 2010;**156**:409-414. e4. DOI: 10.1016/j.jpeds.2009.09.043

[90] Villenave R, Thavagnanam S, Sarlang S, Parker J, Douglas I, Skibinski G, et al. In vitro modeling of respiratory syncytial virus infection of pediatric bronchial epithelium, the primary target of infection in vivo. Proceedings of the National Academy of Sciences of the United States of America. 2012;**109**:5040-5045. DOI: 10.1073/pnas.1110203109

[91] Oshansky CM, Barber JP, Crabtree J, Tripp RA. Respiratory syncytial virus F and G proteins induce interleukin 1alpha, CC, and CXC chemokine responses by normal human bronchoepithelial cells. The Journal of Infectious Diseases. 2010;**201**:1201-1207. DOI: 10.1086/651431

[92] Bueno SM, González PA, Pacheco R, Leiva ED, Cautivo KM, Tobar HE, et al. Host immunity during RSV pathogenesis. International Immunopharmacology. 2008;**8**:1320-1329. DOI: 10.1016/j.intimp.2008.03.012

[93] Jaovisidha P, Peeples ME, Brees AA, Carpenter LR, Moy JN. Respiratory syncytial virus stimulates neutrophil degranulation and chemokine release. Journal of immunology (Baltimore, MD) 1950. 1999;**163**:2816-2820

[94] Becker S, Quay J, Soukup J. Cytokine (tumor necrosis factor, IL-6, and IL-8) production by respiratory syncytial virus-infected human alveolar macrophages. Journal of immunology (Baltimore, MD) 1950. 1991;**147**:4307-4312

[95] Sheeran P, Jafri H, Carubelli C, Saavedra J, Johnson C, Krisher K, et al. Elevated cytokine concentrations in the nasopharyngeal and tracheal secretions of children with respiratory syncytial virus disease. The Pediatric Infectious Disease Journal. 1999;**18**:115-122

[96] Bermejo-Martin JF, Garcia-Arevalo MC, De Lejarazu RO, Ardura J, Eiros JM, Alonso A, et al. Predominance of Th2 cytokines, CXC chemokines and innate immunity mediators at the mucosal level during severe respiratory syncytial virus infection in children. European Cytokine Network. 2007;**18**:162-167. DOI: 10.1684/ecn.2007.0096

[97] Garcia C, Soriano-Fallas A, Lozano J, Leos NB, Gomez AM, Ramilo O, et al. Decreased innate immune cytokine responses correlate with disease severity in children with respiratory syncytial virus and human rhinovirus bronchiolitis. ET Journal. 2012;**31**:86-89. DOI: 10.1097/INF.0b013e31822dc8c1

[98] Díaz PV, Valdivia G, Gaggero AA, Bono MR, Zepeda G, Rivas M, et al. Pro-inflammatory cytokines in nasopharyngeal aspirate from hospitalized children with respiratory syncytial virus infection with or without rhinovirus bronchiolitis, and use of the cytokines as predictors of illness severity. Medicine (Baltimore). 2015;**94**:e1512. DOI: 10.1097/MD.0000000000001512

[99] Garofalo RP, Olszewska-Pazdrak B, Ogra PL, Welliver RC. Beta-chemokines in nasal secretions of infants with respiratory syncytial

virus-induced respiratory infections. Pediatric Asthma, Allergy and Immunology. 2001;**15**:89-96. DOI: 10.1089/088318701753436880

[100] Walsh EE, Peterson DR, Kalkanoglu AE, Lee FE-H, Falsey AR. Viral shedding and immune responses to respiratory syncytial virus infection in older adults. The Journal of Infectious Diseases. 2013;**207**:1424-1432. DOI: 10.1093/infdis/jit038

[101] Hornsleth A, Loland L, Larsen LB. Cytokines and chemokines in respiratory secretion and severity of disease in infants with respiratory syncytial virus (RSV) infection. Journal of Clinical Virology: The Official Publication of the Pan American Society for Clinical Virology. 2001;**21**:163-170

[102] Tian M, Liu F, Wen G, Shi S, Chen R, Zhao D. Effect of variation in RANTES promoter on serum RANTES levels and risk of recurrent wheezing after RSV bronchiolitis in children from Han, Southern China. European Journal of Pediatrics. 2009;**168**:963-967. DOI: 10.1007/s00431-008-0870-3

[103] Hattori S, Shimojo N, Mashimo T, Inoue Y, Ono Y, Kohno Y, et al. Relationship between RANTES polymorphisms and respiratory syncytial virus bronchiolitis in a Japanese infant population. Japanese Journal of Infectious Diseases. 2011;**64**:242-245

[104] Sigurs N, Bjarnason R, Sigurbergsson F. Eosinophil cationic protein in nasal secretion and in serum and myeloperoxidase in serum in respiratory syncytial virus bronchiolitis: Relation to asthma and atopy. Acta Paediatrica (Oslo, Norway: 1992). 1994;**83**:1151-1155

[105] Kim HH, Lee MH, Lee JS. Eosinophil cationic protein and chemokines in nasopharyngeal secretions of infants with respiratory syncytial virus (RSV) bronchiolitis and non-RSV bronchiolitis. Journal of Korean Medical Science. 2007;**22**:37-42. DOI: 10.3346/jkms.2007.22.1.37

[106] Garofalo R, Dorris A, Ahlstedt S, Welliver RC. Peripheral blood eosinophil counts and eosinophil cationic protein content of respiratory secretions in bronchiolitis: Relationship to severity of disease. Pediatric Allergy and Immunology: The Official Publication of the European Society of Pediatric Allergy and Immunology. 1994;**5**:111-117

[107] Brandenburg AH, Groen J, van Steensel-Moll HA, Claas EC, Rothbarth PH, Neijens HJ, et al. Respiratory syncytial virus specific serum antibodies in infants under six months of age: Limited serological response upon infection. Journal of Medical Virology. 1997;**52**:97-104

[108] Kasel JA, Walsh EE, Frank AL, Baxter BD, Taber LH, Glezen WP. Relation of serum antibody to glycoproteins of respiratory syncytial virus with immunity to infection in children. Viral Immunology. 1987;**1**:199-205. DOI: 10.1089/vim.1987.1.199

[109] Nishimura T, Suzue J, Kaji H. Breastfeeding reduces the severity of respiratory syncytial virus infection among young infants: A multi-center prospective study. Pediatrics International (Pediatr Int): Official English Journal of the Japan Pediatric Society. 2009;**51**:812-816. DOI: 10.1111/j.1442-200X.2009.02877.x

[110] Watt PJ, Zardis M, Lambden PR. Age related IgG subclass response to respiratory syncytial virus fusion protein in infected infants. Clinical and Experimental Immunology. 1986;**64**:503-509

[111] Wagner DK, Nelson DL, Walsh EE, Reimer CB, Henderson FW, Murphy BR. Differential immunoglobulin G subclass

antibody titers to respiratory syncytial virus F and G glycoproteins in adults. Journal of Clinical Microbiology. 1987;**25**:748-750

[112] Murphy BR, Graham BS, Prince GA, Walsh EE, Chanock RM, Karzon DT, et al. Serum and nasal-wash immunoglobulin G and A antibody response of infants and children to respiratory syncytial virus F and G glycoproteins following primary infection. Journal of Clinical Microbiology. 1986;**23**:1009-1014

[113] Murphy BR, Alling DW, Snyder MH, Walsh EE, Prince GA, Chanock RM, et al. Effect of age and preexisting antibody on serum antibody response of infants and children to the F and G glycoproteins during respiratory syncytial virus infection. Journal of Clinical Microbiology. 1986;**24**:894-898

[114] Graham BS, Bunton LA, Wright PF, Karzon DT. Reinfection of mice with respiratory syncytial virus. Journal of Medical Virology. 1991;**34**:7-13

[115] Walsh EE, Wang L, Falsey AR, Qiu X, Corbett A, Holden-Wiltse J, et al. Virus-specific antibody, viral load, and disease severity in respiratory syncytial virus infection. The Journal of Infectious Diseases. 2018;**218**:208-217. DOI: 10.1093/infdis/jiy106

[116] Forbes ML, Kumar VR, Yogev R, Wu X, Robbie GJ, Ambrose CS. Serum palivizumab level is associated with decreased severity of respiratory syncytial virus disease in high-risk infants. Human Vaccines and Immunotherapeutics. 2014;**10**:2789-2794. DOI: 10.4161/hv.29635

[117] Hemming VG, Prince GA, Groothuis JR, Siber GR. Hyperimmune globulins in prevention and treatment of respiratory syncytial virus infections. Clinical Microbiology Reviews. 1995;**8**:22-33

[118] Fishaut M, Tubergen D, McIntosh K. Cellular response to respiratory viruses with particular reference to children with disorders of cell-mediated immunity. The Journal of Pediatrics. 1980;**96**:179-186

[119] Cannon MJ, Stott EJ, Taylor G, Askonas BA. Clearance of persistent respiratory syncytial virus infections in immunodeficient mice following transfer of primed T cells. Immunology. 1987;**62**:133-138

[120] Cannon MJ, Openshaw PJ, Askonas BA. Cytotoxic T cells clear virus but augment lung pathology in mice infected with respiratory syncytial virus. The Journal of Experimental Medicine. 1988;**168**:1163-1168. DOI: 10.1084/jem.168.3.1163

[121] Heidema J, Lukens MV, van MWWC, van DMEA, Otten HG, van VAJ, et al. $CD8^+$ T cell responses in Bronchoalveolar lavage fluid and peripheral blood mononuclear cells of infants with severe primary respiratory syncytial virus infections. Journal of Immunology. 2007;**179**:8410-8417. DOI: 10.4049/jimmunol.179.12.8410

[122] Jozwik A, Habibi MS, Paras A, Zhu J, Guvenel A, Dhariwal J, et al. RSV-specific airway resident memory $CD8^+$ T cells and differential disease severity after experimental human infection. Nature Communications. 2015;**6**:10224. DOI: 10.1038/ncomms10224

[123] Kidd P. Th1/Th2 balance: The hypothesis, its limitations, and implications for health and disease. Alternative Medicine Review: A Journal of Clinical Therapeutics. 2003;**8**:223-246

[124] Reithinger R, Dujardin J-C, Louzir H, Pirmez C, Alexander B, Brooker S. Cutaneous leishmaniasis. The Lancet Infectious Diseases. 2007;**7**:581-596. DOI: 10.1016/S1473-3099(07)70209-8

[125] Burke ML, Jones MK, Gobert GN, Li YS, Ellis MK, McManus DP. Immunopathogenesis of human schistosomiasis. Parasite Immunology. 2009;**31**:163-176. DOI: 10.1111/j.1365-3024.2009.01098.x

[126] Everard ML, Swarbrick A, Wrightham M, McIntyre J, Dunkley C, James PD, et al. Analysis of cells obtained by bronchial lavage of infants with respiratory syncytial virus infection. Archives of Disease in Childhood. 1994;**71**:428-432. DOI: 10.1136/adc.71.5.428

[127] Alwan WH, Openshaw PJ. Distinct patterns of T- and B-cell immunity to respiratory syncytial virus induced by individual viral proteins. Vaccine. 1993;**11**:431-437

[128] Alwan WH, Kozlowska WJ, Openshaw PJ. Distinct types of lung disease caused by functional subsets of antiviral T cells. The Journal of Experimental Medicine. 1994;**179**:81-89. DOI: 10.1084/jem.179.1.81

[129] Stack AM, Malley R, Saladino RA, Montana JB, MacDonald KL, Molrine DC. Primary respiratory syncytial virus infection: Pathology, immune response, and evaluation of vaccine challenge strains in a new mouse model. Vaccine. 2000;**18**:1412-1418

[130] Fernández JA, Tapia L, Palomino MA, Larrañaga C, Peña M, Jaramillo H. Plasma interferon-gamma, interleukin-10 and soluble markers of immune activation in infants with primary adenovirus (ADV) and respiratory syncytial virus (RSV) infection. European Cytokine Network. 2005;**16**:35-40

[131] Semple MG, Dankert HM, Ebrahimi B, Correia JB, Booth JA, Stewart JP, et al. Severe respiratory syncytial virus bronchiolitis in infants is associated with reduced airway interferon gamma and substance P. PLoS One. 2007;**2**:e1038. DOI: 10.1371/journal.pone.0001038

[132] Ye Q, Shao W-X, Shang S-Q, Pan Y-X, Shen H-Q, Chen X-J. Epidemiological characteristics and immune status of children with respiratory syncytial virus. Journal of Medical Virology. 2015;**87**:323-329. DOI: 10.1002/jmv.24047

[133] Pinto RA, Arredondo SM, Bono MR, Gaggero AA. Díaz PV. T helper 1/T helper 2 cytokine imbalance in respiratory syncytial virus infection is associated with increased endogenous plasma cortisol. Pediatrics. 2006;**117**:e878-e886. DOI: 10.1542/peds.2005-2119

[134] Bont L, Heijnen CJ, Kavelaars A, van Aalderen WM, Brus F, Draaisma JM, et al. Local interferon-gamma levels during respiratory syncytial virus lower respiratory tract infection are associated with disease severity. The Journal of Infectious Diseases. 2001;**184**:355-358. DOI: 10.1086/322035

[135] Midulla F, Tromba V, Lo Russo L, Mileto F, Sabatino G, Sgarrella M, et al. Cytokines in the nasal washes of children with respiratory syncytial virus bronchiolitis. International Journal of Immunopathology and Pharmacology. 2006;**19**:231-235

[136] Alonso Fernández J, Roine I, Vasquez A, Cáneo M. Soluble interleukin-2 receptor (sCD25) and interleukin-10 plasma concentrations are associated with severity of primary respiratory syncytial virus (RSV) infection. European Cytokine Network. 2005;**16**:81-90

[137] Vieira RA, Diniz EM de A, Ceccon MEJR. Correlation between inflammatory mediators in the nasopharyngeal secretion and in the serum of children with lower respiratory tract infection caused by respiratory syncytial virus and disease severity.

O Jornal Brasileiro de Pneumologia é publicação oficial da Sociedade Brasileira de Pneumologia e Tisiologia. 2010;**36**:59-66

[138] Hassan MA, Eldin AME. Ahmed MM. T-helper2/T-helper1 imbalance in respiratory syncytial virus bronchiolitis in relation to disease severity and outcome. The Egyptian Journal of Immunology. 2008;**15**:153-160

[139] Caballero MT, Serra ME, Acosta PL, Marzec J, Gibbons L, Salim M, et al. TLR4 genotype and environmental LPS mediate RSV bronchiolitis through Th2 polarization. The Journal of Clinical Investigation. 2015;**125**:571-582. DOI: 10.1172/JCI75183

[140] Shalev I, Schmelzle M, Robson SC, Levy G. Making sense of regulatory T cell suppressive function. Seminars in Immunology. 2011;**23**:282-292. DOI: 10.1016/j.smim.2011.04.003

[141] Fulton RB, Meyerholz DK, Varga SM. Foxp3$^+$ CD4 regulatory T cells limit pulmonary immunopathology by modulating the CD8 T cell response during respiratory syncytial virus infection. Journal of Immunology (Baltimore, MD) (1950). 2010;**185**:2382-2392. DOI: 10.4049/jimmunol.1000423

[142] Raiden S, Pandolfi J, Payasliàn F, Anderson M, Rivarola N, Ferrero F, et al. Depletion of circulating regulatory T cells during severe respiratory syncytial virus infection in Young children. American Journal of Respiratory and Critical Care Medicine. 2014;**189**:865-868. DOI: 10.1164/rccm.201311-1977LE

[143] Paramore LC, Ciuryla V, Ciesla G, Liu L. Economic impact of respiratory syncytial virus-related illness in the US. PharmacoEconomics. 2004;**22**:275-284. DOI: 10.2165/00019053-200422050-00001

Section 2

RSV and Late Preterm Infants

Chapter 2

Resolving the Debate on RSV Prophylaxis in Late Preterm Infants

Bosco Paes, Barry Rodgers-Gray and Xavier Carbonell-Estrany

Abstract

There is still active debate in the scientific literature about the importance of providing respiratory syncytial virus (RSV) prophylaxis to late preterm infants born at 33–35 weeks' gestational age (wGA). The American Academy of Pediatrics and the Canadian Paediatric Society position statements only advocate for RSV prophylaxis for infants <30 wGA. Several publications prove the contrary, reporting substantial morbidity and even mortality in older GA infants, following RSV infection. Consequently, other Societies, such as from Spain and Italy, have different criteria, and include as candidates 30–32 wGA infants and 33–35 wGA infants with risk factors for severe RSV disease. This chapter will systematically examine the current evidence for RSV prophylaxis in both early and late preterm infants 29–35 wGA and the cost-effectiveness of this strategy with the use of risk scoring tools. The authors will attempt to reconcile the misconception that late preterm infants do not merit RSV prophylaxis and hopefully resolve the long-standing debate that currently exists in many countries worldwide.

Keywords: respiratory syncytial virus, palivizumab, prematurity, cost effectiveness, prevention, risk scoring tools

1. Introduction

Respiratory syncytial virus (RSV) infection is a common cause of lower respiratory tract infection (LRTI) in young children and is associated with a high global burden of incurred illness. In 2015, 2.8 million new episodes of RSV-related infections were reported in children <5 years of age in high income countries [1]. Of these, at least 383,000 cases required hospital admissions with 3300 accompanying deaths [1]. These figures represent a major healthcare burden, with costs estimated to be $545 million in the United States alone in 2009 [2].

Preterm birth, those born <37 weeks' gestational age (wGA), has been associated with an increased risk for severe RSV-related disease requiring hospitalization (RSVH) [3]. Possible explanations for the increased RSV infection rates in preterm infants are incomplete airway development with reduced alveolar and bronchiolar diameter, increased air space wall thickness, immature immunologic responses, and reduced levels of maternally transmitted, RSV-specific antibodies compared to infants born at term [4]. Globally, about 15 million infants per year are estimated to be born premature, nearly 10% of all births, and thus are at potentially increased risk for RSV infection [5, 6]. Furthermore, the World Health Organization (WHO) reported that the incidence of premature birth is rising [5]. This highlights the importance of preventing RSV-related LRTI and indeed, the WHO has declared the prevention of RSV to be a key healthcare priority [7]. Although several vaccines and antibodies are currently in preclinical or clinical development, it is likely to be several more years before any become commercially available [8, 9]. Therefore, current therapeutic prevention relies solely on palivizumab, a humanized monoclonal antibody, which is indicated for the prevention of RSVH in high-risk infants, such as preterm infants born at ≤35 wGA or those with bronchopulmonary dysplasia (BPD)/chronic lung disease (CLD) or congenital heart disease (CHD) [10, 11]. However, several current guidelines, most notably from the American Academy of Pediatrics (AAP) and the Canadian Pediatric Society, seek to rationalize its use by recommending palivizumab only for infants born at <29 wGA without CLD [12–15], leaving the majority of preterm infants without therapeutic protection.

Risk-scoring tools (RSTs), models to estimate the risk of RSVH based on predetermined risk factors, have been developed to help identify infants at highest risk for RSVH, which may allow for targeted and cost-effective prophylaxis of infants born late preterm [16–19]. Some guidelines, such as those from Spain [20], Italy [21] and Austria [22], advocate the use of such a risk factor-based approach to extend prophylaxis to those preterm infants ≥30 wGA at highest risk.

This chapter aims to provide a rationale for palivizumab prophylaxis in late preterm infants and show that this can be cost effective with the use of validated RSTs.

2. Literature search

A literature review was undertaken using PubMed, EMBASE, and the Cochrane Library of studies including <37 wGA infants without CLD or CHD but with confirmed or probable RSV infection, published between 01 January 1998 and 31 December 2018. To maximize comparability of data, only studies conducted in Western countries, defined as the US, Canada, and Europe (including Turkey and the Russian Federation) were included. The following search terms were used, combined with Medical Subject Headings (MeSH): ["RSV" OR "respiratory syncytial virus" OR "lower respiratory tract infection" OR "LRTI" OR "acute respiratory tract infection" OR "ARTI" OR "ARI" OR "lower respiratory infection (LRI)" OR "bronchiolitis"] AND ["preterm" OR "premature" OR "gestational age" OR "gestation"] AND ["hospitalization*] OR [predisposition" OR "risk factor"] OR ["palivizumab" OR "Synagis" OR "immunoprophylax*" OR "prophylax*"] OR ["cost effective*" OR "Cost"] AND limits: "human, child (birth to 18 years)". Additional publications and reference citations of potential relevance were included as identified by the authors. All original studies, systematic reviews, meta-analyses, and prophylaxis guidelines with at least an English abstract were reviewed.

As this chapter was based solely on published data, ethical approval was not required.

3. Results and discussion

3.1 Literature search

A total of 3532 publications were identified from the literature search, of which 136 were deemed relevant (**Figure 1**). Another 20 references were identified from other sources, resulting in a final number of 156 publications considered during the drafting of this chapter.

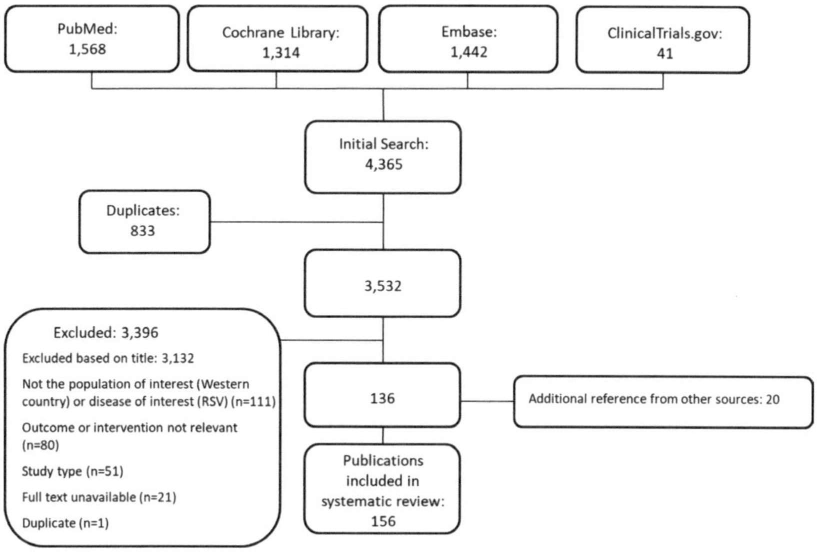

Figure 1.
PRISMA diagram: RSVH in preterm infants (<37 wGA) who received palivizumab.

3.2 What do current guidelines recommend?

There is considerable variation in the published recommendations from national guidelines on the use of palivizumab prophylaxis in preterm infants. The AAP 2014 policy [13, 14], which was unchanged following a review of new evidence in 2017 [15], recommends prophylaxis for healthy preterm infants only if born ≤29 weeks and 0 days (29^0 wGA) and aged <1 year at the start of the RSV season. The justification for this recommendation was partly based on a prospective, population-based surveillance program (n = 2149), undertaken from 2000 to 2005 in the US, which concluded that RSVH rates did not significantly differ between term (≥37 wGA) and preterm (<37 wGA) infants (5.3 vs. 4.6 per 1000 infants, respectively) [23]. Infants born at <30 wGA, on the other hand, experienced a significantly higher RSVH rate of 18.7 per 1000 infants [23]. Further evidence cited was from an analysis of the Tennessee Medicaid database (n = 248,652 infant-years), conducted in the 1990s, which reported higher rates of RSVH in infants <29 wGA compared to term infants with no underlying medical condition [24]. This difference remained consistently higher at up to 23 months of age: 0–5 months, 93.8 vs. 44.1 per 1000 infants; 6–11 months, 46.1 vs. 15.0 per 1000 infants; and, 12–23 months, 30.0 vs. 3.7 per 1000 infants [24]. Another study, which included 1029 ≤ 32 wGA preterm infants, found a decreasing RSVH incidence with increasing GA: ≤26 wGA, 139 per 1000 infants; 27–28 wGA, 99 per 1000 infants; 29–30 wGA, 75 per 1000 infants; and 30–32 wGA, 44 per 1000 infants [25]. Predicated on this evidence, the AAP concluded that the risk of RSVH is considerably higher in those born ≤29° wGA compared to those born between 29^1 and 35^6 wGA and, therefore, prophylaxis should be recommended only in the former [13, 14]. A similar recommendation and rationale is presented in the Canadian RSV position statement, published in 2015 [12]. The Canadian guideline concludes that it is "reasonable but not essential" to offer prophylaxis to infants born <30 wGA who are younger than 6 months at the start of the RSV season, but those born later do not merit prophylaxis, as the magnitude of difference in RSVH incidence between moderate to late preterm infants and infants born at term is not great enough to justify prophylaxis in this group [12]. The authors add that preterm infants are also less vulnerable to RSV infection nowadays due to advances in technology and increased awareness of infection transmission. Preterm infants born >30 wGA are only eligible for prophylaxis if they live in remote regions and would require air transportation for hospitalization [12].

Other guidelines recommend more liberal use of prophylaxis for preterms, with Israeli guidelines, for example, recommending palivizumab for all preterm infants <33 wGA who are aged ≤1 year at the start of the RSV season and 33–35 wGA who are ≤6 months [26]. The Spanish and Italian guidelines recommend prophylaxis for those born between 29 and 31 wGA and aged ≤6 months at the start of the RSV season or if discharged during the season [20, 21]. For 32–35 wGA infants ≤6 months at the start of the RSV season, risk factors predisposing to severe infection and/or need for hospitalization guide the use of prophylaxis [20, 21]. Similar recommendations are reported in a recently published international, expert consensus guideline that guides cost-effective use of prophylaxis for high-risk 32–35 wGA infants with a validated RST [27]. Austrian guidelines have also adopted risk factors to guide prophylaxis for all 29–35 wGA infants, but with a chronological age cut-off of <6 months for 29–32 wGA and <3 months for 33–35 wGA [22].

3.3 Are late preterm infants at increased risk of RSVH compared to term infants?

Many studies in the literature report higher RSVH rates in late preterm infants and children (32–36 wGA) compared to those born at term (**Table 1**) [23, 28–31]. In a Dutch, community-based, cohort study that included 2099 children born between 2002 and 2003 (62 with RSVH), otherwise healthy 32–36 wGA children had a threefold higher RSVH rate compared with full term children (3.9 vs. 1.2%, respectively; relative rate 3.2) [28]. Further evidence comes from a US, retrospective, cohort study involving 599,535 children (7597 admitted for RSVH) that reported a higher RSVH incidence in 33–36 wGA children compared to full term children (12.1 vs. 7.8 per 1000 person-years) [29]. The adjusted hazard ratio for RSVH was 2.45 and 1.92 for children born at 33–34 wGA and 34–36 wGA, respectively [29]. Another US

Study	Number	Age (mo)	EP*	LP*	FT* (≥37 wGA)	Prophylaxed	EP/LP definition (wGA)
Hall 2013 [23]	2149	<24	18.7	6.9	5.3	20%	EP: <30 LP: 32–34
Boyce 2000 [24]	248,652 infant-years	<6	81.8	79.8	44.1	NR	EP: 29–32 LP: 33–35
Stevens 2000 [25]	1029	<12	230	119	NR	NR	EP: <29 MLP: 29–32
Gijtenbeek 2015 [28]	2099	<49	32	39	12	EP: 56.5% MP: 2.2%	EP: <32 LP: 32–36
Helfrich 2015 [29]	599,535	<24	NR	12.1+	7.8+	0%	LP: 33–36
Haerskjold 2015 [30]	421,943	<24	50.8+	28.0+	14.1+	NR	EP: 23–32 LP: 33–35
Cilla 2006 [31]	357	<12	44.2	78.1	1.91	0%	EP: <33 LP: 33–35

**Cases per 1000 infants; +cases per 1000 infant-years; RSVH, respiratory syncytial virus-related hospitalization; EP, early preterm; FT, full term; mo, months; LP, late preterm; MLP, moderate to late preterm; NR, not reported.*

Table 1.
Rates of RSVH.

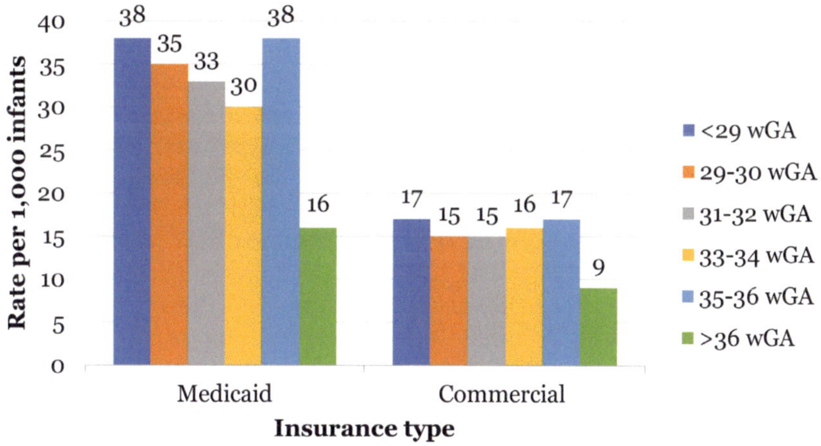

Figure 2.
Rates of RSVH by gestational age group [34]. Hospitalization rates of infants aged less than 1 year at the time of first RSVH in a large American database analysis involving 1,683,188 infants insured via Medicaid and 1,663,832 commercially insured infants [34]. RSVH, respiratory syncytial virus-related hospitalization; wGA, weeks' gestational age.

study, which included 247,566 infants (5322 RSVHs), found that 32–34 wGA infants were at double the risk of RSVH compared to term infants of the same age (odds ratio [OR] 1.94–2.41), and that the risk was highest in the youngest infants [32]. Young age was also associated with an increased risk of RSVH in 32–35 wGA infants in the REPORT study (*n* = 1642) [33]. Interestingly, older age was associated with higher rates of outpatient RSV visits, perhaps related to disease exposure [33]. A Danish database analysis found that, while RSVH incidence decreased with increasing GA, 33–35 wGA children still had a RSVH rate twice as high as full term children (28.0 vs. 14.1 per 1000 years at risk) [30]. Another retrospective study, from Spain, investigating infants born between 1996 and 2000 (*n* = 357), reported a RSVH rate of 44.2 per 1000 children for <33 wGA infants compared to 1.91 per 1000 for ≥38 wGA infants [31]. In this study, 33–35 wGA infants had the highest RSVH rate at 78.1 per 1000 [31].

Other studies have reported that there is not necessarily a simple linear relationship between lower GA and increased risk of RSVH. For example, in a large American database analysis involving 3,347,020 infants, RSVH rates were similar across all gestational age groups from <29 to 36 wGA (**Figure 2**) [34]. In 2016, a systematic review summarizing the evidence from 85 studies undertaken between 1995 and 2015 concluded that, due to considerable variability in methodologies and results, it could not be clearly determined that infants born at younger GAs had higher RSVH rates [3]. Overall, reported RSVH rates were approximately three times higher in premature than term infants, although there was considerable variability across studies (range 1.1–8.1 times higher) [3].

Of potential note, two of the key studies cited by the AAP as evidence to restrict prophylaxis to ≤29° wGA infants reported moderate to late preterm infants to be at high risk of RSVH when considering those aged <6 months [23, 24]. In the US population-based surveillance program [23], the RSVH rate for 32–34 wGA infants ≤5 months of age was 11.0 per 1000 children, compared to a rate of 2.6 per 1000 for those aged 6–23 months. Perhaps more revealing, the Tennessee Medicaid database analysis [24] reported a RSVH rate of 79.8 per 1000 children for 33–35 wGA infants <6 months old compared to 44.1 per 1000 for age-matched, low-risk infants (incidence rate ratio: 1.8, 95% confidence interval [CI]: 1.5–2.1).

3.4 What are the consequences of RSVH in late preterm infants?

The health burden associated with RSVH in late preterm infants has been shown to be substantial [28, 35–38]. A pooled analysis of 7 prospective studies from across the Northern Hemisphere, involving 7820 infants born 33–35 wGA [39–45], reported a median length of stay (LOS) in hospital for RSV of 5.7 days, with 22.2% of infants requiring intensive care unit (ICU) admission for a median of 8.3 days [35]. Supplemental oxygen support was required by 70.4% of cases for a median of 4.9 days and 12.7% required mechanical ventilation for a median of 4.8 days [35]. The US SENTINEL1 study (n = 709) reported a mean RSVH LOS of 5 days with 42% of 29–35 wGA infants being admitted to the ICU (mean ICU LOS: 6 days) [36]. Of those admitted to the ICU, 19% required mechanical ventilation [46]. In a Dutch cohort study [28], the RSV disease burden was found to be similar between <32, 32–36 and 38–42 wGA infants, with no significant differences in terms of hospital LOS (median of 8 vs. 7 vs. 7 days, respectively; $p > 0.3$), oxygen use (82.4 vs. 60.5 vs. 85.7%; $p > 0.1$), mechanical ventilation (5.9 vs. 15.8 vs. 42.9%; $p > 0.1$), or gavage feeding (29.4 vs. 39.5 vs. 42.9%; $p > 0.6$). Other studies, however, have indicated that the disease burden in late preterm infants is higher than in term infants [37, 38]. In a European survey of 3474 infants hospitalized with LRTI [37], while overall LOS in hospital was similar for 33–36 wGA and term infants (mean 11 vs. 9 days, respectively), 33.8% of the former were admitted to the ICU compared to only 14.1% of the latter. The highest disease burden was found in <29 wGA infants (mean LOS 29 days; 54.3% ICU) followed by 29–32 wGA infants (mean 24 days; 48.8% ICU) [37]. A retrospective US study [38], involving 215 term infants and 89 infants <37 wGA, reported that 33–35 wGA infants had the highest rate of intubation (38.7 vs. ≤32 wGA: 21.4% vs. 36 wGA: 20.0 vs. ≥37 wGA: 12.1%; $p = 0.002$) and longest hospital LOS (mean 8.4 vs. 6.8 vs. 4.9 vs. 4.1 days; $p < 0.0001$) and ICU LOS (mean 7.7 vs. 5.8 vs. 4.2 vs. 3.8 days; $p = 0.021$) compared with infants in other GA groups.

As a consequence of RSVH, preterm infants may develop longer-term morbidities, such as recurrent wheezing [47–51]. In the SPRING study, a multicenter, observational, nested, case–control study undertaken in Spain, 32–35 wGA infants with RSVH (n = 125) had a significantly higher incidence of recurrent wheezing through the first 6 years of life, independent of familial or childhood atopy, compared to infants born at the same GA without RSVH (n = 362) (66.7 vs. 49.2%, respectively; $p = 0.001$) [47]. While current wheezing rates remained higher in cases than controls each year, the difference remained significant only until 3 years old. Allied to this, respiratory-related quality of life was significantly lower in RSVH cases than controls (TAPQOL: 93.96 vs. 95.76, respectively; $p = 0.001$). Hospital resource use through 6 years of life was also higher in RSVH cases than controls (outpatient services: 84.0 vs. 66.3%, respectively, $p < 0.001$; emergency care: 62.4 vs. 33.7%, $p < 0.001$). Further analysis revealed that RSVH was the single most important factor for recurrent wheezing (OR: 4.40; $p < 0.001$) [47]. Similar results have been reported in the Dutch RISK study [51]. At the 6-year follow-up of this birth cohort of 2210 32–35 wGA infants, the current wheezing rate was 27.7% for RSVH cases and 17.6% for non-hospitalized infants (OR: 1.8; 95% CI: 1.11–2.85). RSVH was found to be an independent risk factor for current wheezing at 6 years in children without atopic predisposition (OR: 4.1; 95% CI: 1.22–12.52) [51]. Other studies have reported higher healthcare resource utilization (including emergency department visits, outpatient visits, and hospitalizations) in late preterm infants in the year following RSV LRTI compared to their counterparts without such an infection [52, 53].

3.5 How effective is palivizumab prophylaxis in late preterm infants?

Palivizumab has proven effective in late preterm infants, reducing the incidence of RSVH by up to 82% in prospective, comparative studies (**Table 2**) [8, 10, 11, 39, 54]. A *post-hoc* analysis of the pivotal IMpact study, a randomized clinical trial including 724 preterm infants, showed the effectiveness of palivizumab to be similar in <29 wGA and 32–35 wGA infants (relative risk reduction: 80.4 vs. 82.1%, respectively) [11]. The Spanish FLIP-2 study, which reported a 68.3% reduction in RSVH with prophylaxis, found that not receiving palivizumab was an independent risk factor for RSVH (OR: 0.25; 95% CI: 0.13–0.49) in 32–35 wGA infants [39]. Registry data have confirmed the efficacy of palivizumab, with the Palivizumab Outcomes Registry from the US reporting RSVH rates of 0.2–1.6% in 32–35 wGA infants across four RSV seasons (2000–2004) [55], compared to 10.1% in the placebo arm of the IMpact trial [11]. Similar results were seen in the Canadian Registry of Palivizumab (CARESS) [56], with a RSVH incidence of 1.4% in 33–35 wGA infants during the 2006–2011 RSV seasons, compared to 8.2% (untreated subjects) in the IMpact study [11]. A propensity score weighted regression analysis based on a prospective, international trial ($n = 849$), showed that palivizumab prophylaxis significantly reduced RSVHs by 74.1% in 29–35 wGA infants, without comorbidities, aged ≤6 months [57].

Some studies have indicated that restricting palivizumab to ≤29 wGA infants does not increase the overall RSVH rate in children <2 years, while saving money on palivizumab prescriptions [58, 59]. A retrospective US study reported no difference in RSVH rates following introduction of the AAP 2014 policy (pre: 5.37/1000 vs. post: 5.78/1000; $p = 0.622$) [58]. Similar results were reported in Italy following introduction of the same policy in 2016, with the RSVH rate being 6.3/1000 before implementation and 5.5/1000 afterwards [59]. Other studies, however, have reported RSVH rates to have increased by up to 103% following implementation of a more restrictive policy [60–63].

Several studies have indicated that, by preventing RSV infection, palivizumab can reduce subsequent wheezing in premature children, including those born late preterm [48, 54, 64–66]. In the MAKI study, a randomized, placebo-controlled trial of palivizumab that included 429 infants born at 32–35 wGA, the proportion of children with wheezing was reduced by 41.9% in the palivizumab group at 6 years (11.6 vs. 19.9% for placebo) [48]. Similar results were seen in the Japanese CREW study ($n = 444$; 349 received palivizumab ≤1 year), where recurrent wheezing was significantly lower in palivizumab-treated, 33–35 wGA infants than chronologically age-matched untreated infants (15.3 vs. 31.6%, respectively; $p = 0.003$) [65].

Study	Number	Gestational age group	RSVH incidence		RRR (%)
			Palivizumab	Untreated	
Notario 2014 [11]	724	32–35 wGA	1.8%	10.1%	82.1%
		33–35 wGA	2.2%	8.2%	73.2%
MAKI study, Blanken 2013 [54]	429	33–35 wGA	0.9%	5.1%	82.4%
FLIP-2 study, Figueras-Aloy 2008 [39]	5441	32–35 wGA	1.3%	4.1%	68.3%

RRR: relative risk reduction; RSVH: Respiratory-syncytial-virus-related hospitalization; wGA: weeks' gestational age.

Table 2.
Prospective, comparative studies on the effectiveness of palivizumab prophylaxis in reducing RSVH in late preterm infants.

3.6 Can the use of risk factors target infants at highest risk for RSV infection and improve the cost-effectiveness of prophylaxis in the late preterm population?

A key argument for restricting the use of palivizumab to <29 wGA infants is cost-effectiveness. Late preterm infants represent approximately 85% of preterm births [6], and it is unrealistic that prophylaxis of all these infants would ever be cost-effective. For this reason, the use of risk factors, to identify infants at the highest risk of RSVH, appears a pragmatic approach. There have been several RSTs developed and validated, including those in Canada [17], Spain [18], and the Netherlands [41]. Recently, a RST, involving 32–35 wGA infants, was published using pooled, individual patient data (n = 13,475) from six prospective, observational studies across the Northern Hemisphere [16], which included Canada [40], Italy [42], the Netherlands [41], Spain [39], the US [44], and a multinational cohort comprising subjects from Europe, the Middle East, North America, and Asia [45]. The RST was externally validated against a further study from Ireland (n = 1078) [43]. The RST includes three risk factors: birth 3 months before and 2 months after the RSV season start date; smokers in the household and/or smoking during pregnancy; and siblings (excluding multiples) and/or (planned) day-care (**Figure 3**) [16]. Predictive accuracy was demonstrated to be good, with an area under the receiver operating characteristic curve (AUROC) of 0.773, and sensitivity/specificity of 68.9 and 73.0%, respectively. The RST provides cut-off scores for infants at low- (≤19; 1.0% RSVH rate), moderate- (20–45; 3.3%), and high-risk (50–56; 9.5%) for RSVH [16].

The cost-effectiveness of using the multinational RST has not been formally assessed; however, economic evaluations have been undertaken on the use of other RSTs or risk-factor based approaches to targeting prophylaxis in late preterm 33–35 wGA infants [19, 67, 68]. The Canadian RST, based on data from the PICNIC study [40], included seven variables: small for GA (<10th percentile); male sex; born early during the RSV season (November, December, January); family history without eczema; subject or siblings in daycare; >5 individuals in the home, including the subject; and, >1 smoker in the household [17]. The AUROC was 0.762 and sensitivity and specificity were 68.2 and 71.9%, respectively. The RST included cut-off scores of 0–48, 49–64, and 65–100 for low-, moderate-, and high-risk infants, respectively

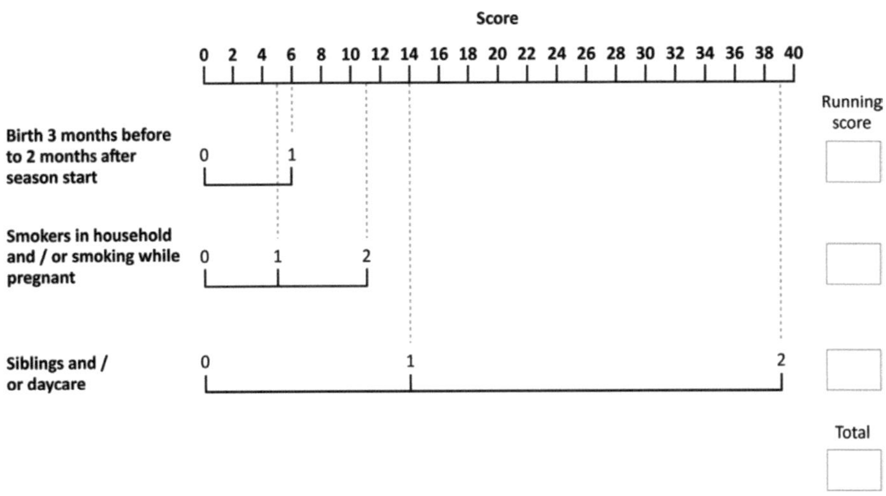

Figure 3.
Risk factor scoring tool for late preterm infants [16]. 0 = No/Not Present; 1 = Yes/Present for one risk factor; 2 = Yes/Present for both risk factors. Score—Low-risk: ≤19; Moderate-risk: 20–45; High-risk: 50–56.

[17]. A cost-effective analysis from 2008, using a decision analytic model, reported incremental cost-effectiveness ratios (ICERs) of CDN$179,699, CDN$34,215, and CDN$5765 per quality-adjusted life year (QALY) for low-, moderate-, and high-risk infants, respectively; the ICERs for moderate- and high-risk infants were considered cost-effective under the Canadian healthcare system (medications commonly adopted with ICERs per QALY of CDN$50–75,000 at that time) [19]. The Dutch RST was based on data from the RISK study and included four variables: family atopy; birth Aug-14 to Dec-01; breastfeeding; and siblings or daycare attendance [41]. The AUROC was 0.703 and the cut-off score for low-risk was defined as <16 (3.5% RSVH rate) and for high-risk as ≥16 (10.0% RSVH rate) [41]. Assuming all high-risk infants would receive prophylaxis, a decision model analysis produced an ICER of €214,748 per QALY, for moderately preterm infants 32–35 wGA, which was considered not cost-effective at a threshold of €80,000 per QALY [67]. Another analysis on 33–35 wGA infants, using data from the Spanish FLIP-2 study [39], assessed cost-effectiveness based on infants having either 2 major risk factors and 2 minor risk factors (group A), 2 major and 1 minor risk factors (B), or 2 major risk factors (C) [68]. Major risk factors included chronological age < 10 weeks at the start of the RSV season or being born during the first 10 weeks of the season, school-age siblings or daycare attendance; whereas minor risk factors included maternal smoking during pregnancy and male sex [69]. Again using a decision analytic model, the incremental cost-utility ratio of €11,550.37, €14,177.18 and €13,937.61 per QALY gained for groups A, B and C, respectively, were derived and were deemed all highly cost-effective based on a threshold of €30,000 per QALY from both a National Health System and societal perspective [68]. An Austrian analysis reported palivizumab prophylaxis to be cost-effective in 33–35 wGA infants at €21,862 per QALY from the healthcare system perspective, when administered to those <3 months of age with risk factors [70]. It is important to note that the Canadian, Spanish and Austrian analyses modeled the effects of long-term respiratory morbidity, using life-time (Canadian and Austrian) and 6-year time horizons (Spanish), while the Dutch study included follow-up to only 1 year of age [19, 67, 68, 70]. This could, in part, account for the differences in cost-effectiveness reported. It would be interesting to see the impact on the ICERs if the increased rates of wheezing in children with a history of RSVH at 6 years in the RISK study (27.7 vs. 17.6% for non-hospitalized) were incorporated into the Dutch cost-effectiveness analysis. The ICERs reported from all three studies reflect costs from the healthcare system or payer perspective; including the societal impact of RSVH could potentially reduce the ICERs by 15–40% [19, 68]. The models also do not include the impact of RSV in the community setting, which could reduce the ICERs still further.

4. Conclusion

There is a sizable body of evidence demonstrating that late preterm infants are at increased risk of RSVH, resulting in substantial morbidity, both in terms of acute hospitalization and longer-term respiratory sequelae. While we await the availability of a safe and effective vaccine or a newer monoclonal antibody with an extended half-life, palivizumab remains the only proven therapy for reducing the incidence of RSVH in late preterm infants, and may also reduce subsequent wheezing. The use of RSTs and risk factors provides a mechanism to cost-effectively target the most vulnerable of these infants to receive palivizumab. It is recommended that countries adopt the multinational RST (**Figure 3**) and adapt this with local data and cut-offs, as available, to meet country-specific requirements and available funding.

Acknowledgements

This chapter is the independent views of the authors. No funding was received for developing this chapter.

Conflict of interest

Xavier Carbonell-Estrany has acted as expert advisor and speaker for AbbVie and has received honoraria for this. Bosco Paes has received research funding and compensation as advisor and lecturer from AbbVie Corporation. Barry Rodgers-Gray is an employee of Strategen; Strategen has received fees for work on various projects for AbbVie. The authors have no other conflict of interest to declare.

Author details

Bosco Paes[1], Barry Rodgers-Gray[2] and Xavier Carbonell-Estrany[3]*

1 Neonatal Division, Department of Pediatrics, McMaster University, Hamilton, Canada

2 Strategen Limited, Basingstoke, UK

3 Neonatology Service, Hospital Clinic, Institut d'Investigacions Biomediques August Pi Suñer, Barcelona, Spain

*Address all correspondence to: carbonell@comb.cat

References

[1] Shi T, McAllister DA, O'Brien KL, Simoes EAF, Madhi SA, Gessner BD, et al. Global, regional, and national disease burden estimates of acute lower respiratory infections due to respiratory syncytial virus in young children in 2015: A systematic review and modelling study. Lancet. 2017;**390**:946-958. DOI: 10.1016/S0140-6736(17)30938-8

[2] Hasegawa K, Tsugawa Y, Brown DF, Mansbach JM, Camargo CA Jr. Trends in bronchiolitis hospitalizations in the United States, 2000-2009. Pediatrics. 2013;**132**:28-36. DOI: 10.1542/peds.2012-3877

[3] Figueras-Aloy J, Manzoni P, Paes B, Simões EA, Bont L, Checchia PA, et al. Defining the risk and associated morbidity and mortality of severe respiratory syncytial virus infection among preterm infants without chronic lung disease or congenital heart disease. Infectious Disease and Therapy. 2016;**5**:417-452. DOI: 10.1007/s40121-016-0130-1

[4] Resch B. Respiratory syncytial virus infection in high-risk infants—An update on palivizumab prophylaxis. Open Microbiology Journal. 2014;**11**:71-77. DOI: 10.2174/1874285801408010071

[5] World Health Organization. Born too soon: The global action report on preterm birth [Internet]. 2012. Available from: http://apps.who.int/iris/bitstream/10665/44864/1/9789241503433_eng.pdf?ua=1 [Accessed: 2019-01-24]

[6] Martin JA, Hamilton BE, Osterman MJK, Driscoll AK, Mathews TJ. Births: Final data for 2015. National Vital Statistics Reports. 2017;**66**:1-69

[7] Modjarrad K, Giersing B, Kaslow DC, Smith PG, Moorthy VS, WHO RSV vaccine consultation expert group. WHO consultation on respiratory syncytial virus vaccine development report from a World Health Organization meeting held on 23-24 March 2015. Vaccine. 2016;**34**:190-197. DOI: 10.1016/j.vaccine.2015.05.093

[8] Simoes EAF, Bont L, Manzoni P, Fauroux B, Paes B, Figueras-Aloy J, et al. Past, present and future approaches to the prevention and treatment of respiratory syncytial virus infection in children. Infectious Disease and Therapy. 2018;**7**:87-120. DOI: 10.1007/s40121-018-0188-z

[9] Mazur NI, Martinon-Torres F, Baraldi E, Fauroux B, Greenough A, Heikkinen T, et al. Lower respiratory tract infection caused by respiratory syncytial virus: Current management and new therapeutics. The Lancet Respiratory Medicine. 2015;**3**:888-900. DOI: 10.1016/S2213-2600(15)00255-6

[10] The IMpact-RSV Study Group. Palivizumab, a humanized respiratory syncytial virus monoclonal antibody, reduces hospitalization from respiratory syncytial virus infection in high-risk infants. Pediatrics. 1998;**102**:531-537

[11] Notario G, Vo P, Gooch K, Deaton R, Wu X, Harris B. Respiratory syncytial virus-related hospitalization in premature infants without bronchopulmonary dysplasia: Subgroup efficacy analysis of the IMpact-RS V trial by gestational age group. Pediatric Health, Medicine and Therapeutics. 2014;**5**:43-48. DOI: 10.2147/PHMT.S59572

[12] Robinson JL, Le Saux N, Canadian Paediatric Society, Infectious Diseases and Immunization Committee. Preventing hospitalizations for respiratory syncytial virus infection. Paediatrics & Child Health. 2015;**20**:321-333. DOI: 10.1093/pch/20.6.321

[13] American Academy of Pediatrics Committee on Infectious Diseases, American Academy of Pediatrics Bronchiolitis Guidelines Committee. Updated guidance for palivizumab prophylaxis among infants and young children at increased risk of hospitalization for respiratory syncytial virus infection. Pediatrics. 2014;**134**:415-420. DOI: 10.1542/peds.2014-1665

[14] American Academy of Pediatrics Committee on Infectious Diseases. Updated guidance for palivizumab prophylaxis among infants and young children at increased risk of hospitalization for respiratory syncytial virus infection. Pediatrics. 2014;**134**:e620-e638. DOI: 10.1542/peds.2014-1666

[15] Munoz FM, Ralston SL, Meissner HC. RSV recommendations unchanged after review of new data. AAP News. 2017;**38**:1-4

[16] Blanken MO, Bosco P, Anderson EJ, Lanari M, Sheridan-Pereira M, Buchan S, et al. Risk scoring tool to predict respiratory syncytial virus hospitalisation in premature infants. Pediatric Pulmonology. 2018;**53**: 605-612. DOI: 10.1002/ppul.23960

[17] Sampalis JS, Langley J, Carbonell-Estrany X, Paes B, O'Brien K, Allen U, et al. Development and validation of a risk scoring tool to predict respiratory syncytial virus hospitalization in premature infants born at 33 through 35 completed weeks of gestation. Medical Decision Making. 2008;**28**:471-480. DOI: 10.1177/0272989X08315238

[18] Simoes EA, Carbonell-Estrany X, Fullarton JR, Liese JG, Figueras-Aloy J, Doering G, et al. A predictive model for respiratory syncytial virus (RSV) hospitalisation of premature infants born at 33-35 weeks of gestational age, based on data from the Spanish FLIP study. Respiratory Research. 2008;(9):78. DOI: 10.1186/1465-9921-9-78

[19] Lanctot KL, Masoud ST, Paes BA, Tarride JE, Chiu A, Hui C, et al. The cost-effectiveness of palivizumab for respiratory syncytial virus prophylaxis in premature infants with a gestational age of 32-35 weeks: A Canadianbased analysis. Current Medical Research and Opinion. 2008;**24**:3223-3237. DOI: 10.1185/03007990802484234

[20] Figueras Aloy J, Carbonell Estrany X, Comité de Estándares de la SENeo. Actualización de las recomendaciones de la Sociedad Española de Neonatología Para la utilización del palivizumab Como profilaxis de las infecciones graves por el virus respiratorio sincitial. Anales de Pediatría. 2015;**82**:199e1-199e2

[21] Bollani L, Baraldi E, Chirico G, Dotta A, Lanari M, Del Vecchio A, et al. Revised recommendations concerning palivizumab prophylaxis for respiratory syncytial virus (RSV). Italian Journal of Pediatrics. 2015;**41**:97. DOI: 10.1186/s13052-015-0203-x

[22] Resch B. Respiratory syncytial virus (RSV) prophylaxis: Summary of the Austrian recommendations [German]. Pädiatrie Pädologie. 2009;**2**:35-36

[23] Hall CB, Weinberg GA, Blumkin AK, Edwards KM, Staat MA, Schultz AF, et al. Respiratory syncytial virus-associated hospitalizations among children less than 24 months of age. Pediatrics. 2013;**132**:e341-e348. DOI: 10.1542/peds.2013-0303

[24] Boyce TG, Mellen BG, Mitchel EF Jr, Wright PF, Griffin MR. Rates of hospitalization for respiratory syncytial virus infection among children in Medicaid. The Journal of Pediatrics. 2000;**137**:865-870. DOI: 10.1067/mpd.2000.110531

[25] Stevens TP, Sinkin RA, Hall CB, Maniscalco WM, McConnochie KM.

Respiratory syncytial virus and premature infants born at 32 weeks' gestation or earlier: Hospitalization and economic implications of prophylaxis. Archives of Pediatrics & Adolescent Medicine. 2000;**154**:55-61. DOI: 10-1001/pubs

[26] Slezinger Y. The Committee's Recommendations on Behalf of the Israeli Association of Pediatrics of Indications for Respiratory Syncytial Virus Passive Immunization. Jerusalem: Israeli Association of Pediatrics; 2014

[27] Sanchez-Luna M, Manzoni P, Paes B, Baraldi E, Cossey V, Kugelmang A, et al. Expert consensus on palivizumab use for respiratory syncytial virus in developed countries. Paediatric Respiratory Reviews. DOI: 10.1016/j.prrv.2018.12.001

[28] Gijtenbeek RG, Kerstjens JM, Reijneveld SA, Duiverman EJ, Bos AF, Vrijlandt EJ. RSV infection among children born moderately preterm in a community-based cohort. European Journal of Pediatrics. 2015;**174**:435-442. DOI: 10.1007/s00431-014-2415-2

[29] Helfrich AM, Nylund CM, Eberly MD, Eide MB, Stagliano DR. Healthy late-preterm infants born 33-36 weeks gestational age have higher risk for respiratory syncytial virus hospitalization. Early Human Development. 2015;**91**:541-546. DOI: 10.1016/j.earlhumdev.2015.06.009

[30] Haerskjold A, Kristensen K, Kamper-Jorgensen M, Nybo Andersen AM, Ravn H, Stensballe LG. Risk factors for hospitalization for respiratory syncytial virus infection: A population-based cohort study of Danish children. The Pediatric Infectious Disease Journal. 2016;**35**:61-65. DOI: 10.1097/INF.0000000000000924

[31] Cilla G, Sarasua A, Montes M, Arostegui N, Vicente D, Perez-Yarza E, et al. Risk factors for hospitalization due to respiratory syncytial virus infection among infants in the Basque Country, Spain. Epidemiology and infection. 2006;**134**:506-513. DOI: 10.1017/S0950268805005571

[32] Winterstein AG, Knox CA, Kubilis P, Hampp C. Appropriateness of age thresholds for respiratory syncytial virus immunoprophylaxis in moderate-preterm infants: A cohort study. JAMA Pediatrics. 2013;**167**:1118-1124. DOI: 10.1001/jamapediatrics.2013.2636

[33] Simoes EA, Anderson EJ, Wu X, Ambrose CS. Effects of chronologic age and young child exposure on respiratory syncytial virus disease among US preterm infants born at 32 to 35 weeks gestation. PLoS ONE. 2016;**11**:e0166226. DOI: 10.1371/journal.pone.0166226

[34] McLaurin KK, Farr AM, Wade SW, Diakun DR, Stewart DL. Respiratory syncytial virus hospitalization outcomes and costs of full-term and preterm infants. Journal of Perinatology. 2016;**36**:990-996. DOI: 10.1038/jp.2016.113

[35] Anderson EJ, Carbonell-Estrany X, Blanken M, Lanari M, Sheridan-Pereira M, Rodgers-Gray B, et al. Burden of severe respiratory syncytial virus disease among 33-35 weeks' gestational age infants born during multiple respiratory syncytial virus seasons. The Pediatric Infectious Disease Journal. 2017;**36**:160-167. DOI: 10.1097/INF.0000000000001377

[36] Anderson EJ, Krilov LR, DeVincenzo JP, Checchia PA, Halasa N, Simoes EA, et al. SENTINEL1: An observational study of respiratory syncytial virus hospitalizations among U.S. infants born at 29 to 35 weeks' gestational age not receiving immunoprophylaxis. American Journal of Perinatology. 2017;**34**:51-61. DOI: 10.1055/s-0036-1584147

[37] Van de Steen O, Miri F, Gunjaca M, Klepac V, Gross B, Notario G, et al. The burden of severe respiratory

syncytial virus disease among children younger than 1 year in central and Eastern Europe. Infectious Disease and Therapy. 2016;**5**:125-137. DOI: 10.1007/s40121-016-0109-y

[38] Horn SD, Smout RJ. Effect of prematurity on respiratory syncytial virus hospital resource use and outcomes. The Journal of Pediatrics. 2003;**143**:S133-S141. DOI: 10.1067/S0022-3476(03)00509-2

[39] Figueras-Aloy J, Carbonell-Estrany X, Quero-Jimenez J, Fernandez-Colomer B, Guzman-Cabanas J, Echaniz-Urcelay I, et al. FLIP-2 study: Risk factors linked to respiratory syncytial virus infection requiring hospitalization in premature infants born in Spain at a gestational age of 32 to 35 weeks. The Pediatric Infectious Disease Journal. 2008;**27**:788-793. DOI: 10.1097/INF.0b013e3181710990

[40] Law BJ, Langley JM, Allen U, Paes B, Lee DS, Mitchell M, et al. The Pediatric investigators collaborative network on infections in Canada study of predictors of hospitalization for respiratory syncytial virus infection for infants born at 33 through 35 completed weeks of gestation. The Pediatric Infectious Disease Journal. 2004;**23**:806-814. DOI: 10.1097/01.inf.0000137568.71589.bd

[41] Blanken MO, Koffijberg H, Nibbelke EE, Rovers MM, Bont L, Dutch RSV Neonatal Network. Prospective validation of a prognostic model for respiratory syncytial virus bronchiolitis in late preterm infants: A multicenter birth cohort study. PLoS ONE. 2013;**8**:e59161. DOI: 10.1371/journal.pone.0059161

[42] Lanari M, Prinelli F, Adorni F, Di Santo S, Vandini S, Silvestri M, et al. Risk factors for bronchiolitis hospitalization during the first year of life in a multicentre Italian birth cohort. Italian Journal of Pediatrics. 2015;**41**:40. DOI: 10.1186/s13052-015-0149-z

[43] Sheridan-Pereira M, Murphy J, Sloan J, Crispino G, Leahy A, Corcoran JD, et al. Respiratory syncytial virus preterm (32-36 completed weeks of gestation) risk estimation measure for RSV hospitalization in Ireland: A prospective study. The Pediatric Infectious Disease Journal. 2016;**35**:19-24. DOI: 10.1097/INF.0000000000000918

[44] Ambrose CS, Anderson EJ, Simoes EA, Wu X, Elhefni H, Park CL, et al. Respiratory syncytial virus disease in preterm infants in the U.S. born at 32-35 weeks gestation not receiving immunoprophylaxis. The Pediatric Infectious Disease Journal. 2014;**33**:576-582. DOI: 10.1097/INF.0000000000000219

[45] Stranak Z, Saliba E, Kosma P, Posfay-Barbe K, Yunis K, Farstad T, et al. Predictors of RSV LRTI hospitalization in infants born at 33 to 35 weeks gestational age: A large multinational study (PONI). PLoS ONE. 2016;**11**:e0157446. DOI: 10.1371/journal.pone.0157446

[46] De Vincenzo J. A multicenter observational study of respiratory syncytial virus hospitalizations among US infants born at 29-35 weeks' gestational age not receiving immunoprophylaxis in 2014-2016. In: Presented at Pediatric Academic Societies (PAS) Annual Meeting; May 6-9, 2017; San Francisco, CA, Session SFC-2004: Abstract #3560.8. 2017

[47] Carbonell-Estrany X, Perez-Yarza EG, Garcia LS, Guzman Cabanas JM, Boria EV, Atienza BB, et al. Long-term burden and respiratory effects of respiratory syncytial virus hospitalization in preterm infants-the SPRING study. PLoS ONE. 2015;**10**:e0125422. DOI: 10.1371/journal.pone.0125422

[48] Scheltema NM, Nibbelke EE, Pouw J, Blanken MO, Rovers MM, Naaktgeboren CA, et al. Respiratory

syncytial virus prevention and asthma in healthy preterm infants: A randomised controlled trial. The Lancet Respiratory Medicine. 2018;**6**:257-264. DOI: 10.1016/S2213-2600(18)30055-9

[49] Drysdale SB, Lo J, Prendergast M, Alcazar M, Wilson T, Zuckerman M, et al. Lung function of preterm infants before and after viral infections. European Journal of Pediatrics. 2014;**173**:1497-1504. DOI: 10.1007/s00431-014-2343-1

[50] Greenough A, Broughton S. Chronic manifestations of respiratory syncytial virus infection in premature infants. The Pediatric Infectious Disease Journal. 2005;**24**:S184-S187

[51] Korsten K, Blanken MO, Buiteman BJM, Nibbelke EE, Naaktgeboren CA, Bont LJ, et al. RSV hospitalization in infancy increases the risk of current wheeze at age 6 in late preterm born children without atopic predisposition. European Journal of Pediatrics. [Epub ahead of print]. DOI: 10.1007/s00431-018-03309-0

[52] Palmer L, Hall CB, Katkin JP, Shi N, Masaquel AS, McLaurin KK, et al. Respiratory outcomes, utilization and costs 12 months following a respiratory syncytial virus diagnosis among commercially insured late-preterm infants. Current Medical Research and Opinion. 2011;**27**:403-412. DOI: 10.1185/03007995.2010.542744

[53] Sampalis JS. Morbidity and mortality after RSV-associated hospitalizations among premature Canadian infants. The Journal of Pediatrics. 2003;**143**:S150-S156. DOI: 10.1067/S0022-3476(03)00513-4

[54] Blanken MO, Rovers MM, Molenaar JM, Winkler-Seinstra PL, Meijer A, Kimpen JL, et al. Respiratory syncytial virus and recurrent wheeze in healthy preterm infants. The New England Journal of Medicine. 2013;**368**:1791-1799. DOI: 10.1056/NEJMoa1211917

[55] Frogel M, Nerwen C, Cohen A, VanVeldhuisen P, Harrington M, Boron M, et al. Prevention of hospitalization due to respiratory syncytial virus: Results from the palivizumab outcomes registry. Journal of Perinatology. 2008;**28**:511-517. DOI: 10.1038/jp.2008.28

[56] Paes B, Mitchell I, Li A, Lanctot KL, CARESS investigators. A comparative study of respiratory syncytial virus (RSV) prophylaxis in premature infants within the Canadian registry of palivizumab (CARESS). European Journal of Clinical Microbiology & Infectious Diseases. 2012;**31**:2703-2711. DOI: 10.1007/s10096-012-1617-7

[57] Anderson EJ, Carosone-Link P, Yogev R, Yi J, Simoes EAF. Effectiveness of palivizumab in high-risk infants and children: A propensity score weighted regression analysis. The Pediatric Infectious Disease Journal. 2017;**36**:699-704. DOI: 10.1097/INF.0000000000001533

[58] Grindeland CJ, Mauriello CT, Leedahl DD, Richter LM, Meyer AC. Association between updated guideline-based palivizumab administration and hospitalizations for respiratory syncytial virus infections. The Pediatric Infectious Disease Journal. 2016;**35**:728-732. DOI: 10.1097/INF.0000000000001150

[59] Belleudi V, Trotta F, Pinnarelli L, Davoli M, Addis A. Neonatal outcomes following new reimbursement limitations on palivizumab in Italy. Archives of Disease in Childhood. 2018;**103**(12):1163-1167. DOI: 10.1136/archdischild-2018-315349

[60] Rajah B, Sánchez PJ, Garcia-Maurino C, Leber A, Ramilo O, Mejias A. Impact of the updated guidance for palivizumab prophylaxis against respiratory syncytial virus infection: A

single center experience. The Journal of Pediatrics. 2017;**181**:183e1-188e1. DOI: 10.1016/j.jpeds.2016.10.074

[61] Kong AM, Krilov LR, Fergie J, Goldstein M, Diakun D, Wade SW, et al. The 2014-2015 National Impact of the 2014 American Academy of Pediatrics guidance for respiratory syncytial virus Immunoprophylaxis on preterm infants born in the United States. American Journal of Perinatology. 2018;**35**: 192-200. DOI: 10.1055/s-0037-1606352

[62] Capizzi A, Silvestri M, Orsi A, Cutrera R, Rossi GA, Sacco O. The impact of the recent AAP changes in palivizumab authorization on RSV-induced bronchiolitis severity and incidence. Italian Journal of Pediatrics. 2017;**43**:71. DOI: 10.1186/s13052-017-0390-8

[63] Blake SM, Tanaka D, Bendz LM, Staebler S, Brandon D. Evaluation of the financial and health burden of infants at risk for respiratory syncytial virus. Advances in Neonatal Care. 2017;**17**:292-298. DOI: 10.1097/ANC.0000000000000367

[64] Yoshihara S, Kusuda S, Mochizuki H, Okada K, Nishima S, Simoes EA, et al. Effect of palivizumab prophylaxis on subsequent recurrent wheezing in preterm infants. Pediatrics. 2013;**132**:811-818. DOI: 10.1542/peds.2013-0982

[65] Mochizuki H, Kusuda S, Okada K, Yoshihara S, Furuya H, Simoes EAF, et al. Palivizumab prophylaxis in preterm infants and subsequent recurrent wheezing. Six-year follow-up study. American Journal of Respiratory and Critical Care Medicine. 2017;**196**:29-38. DOI: 10.1164/rccm.201609-1812OC

[66] Simoes EA, Groothuis JR, Carbonell-Estrany X, Rieger CH, Mitchell I, Fredrick LM, et al. Palivizumab prophylaxis, respiratory syncytial virus, and subsequent recurrent wheezing. The Journal of Pediatrics. 2007;**151**:34-42. DOI: 10.1016/j.jpeds.2007.02.032

[67] Blanken MO, Frederix GW, Nibbelke EE, Koffijberg H, Sanders EAM, Rovers MM, et al. Cost-effectiveness of rule-based immunoprophylaxis against respiratory syncytial virus infections in preterm infants. European Journal of Pediatrics. 2018;**177**:133-144. DOI: 10.1007/s00431-017-3046-1

[68] Sanchez-Luna M, Burgos-Pol R, Oyagüez I, Figueras-Aloy J, Sanchez-Solis M, Martinon-Torres F, et al. Cost-utility analysis of palivizumab for respiratory syncytial virus infection prophylaxis in preterm infants: Update based on the clinical evidence in Spain. BMC Infectious Diseases. 2017;**17**:687. DOI: 10.1186/s12879-017-2803-0

[69] Figueras-Aloy J, Carbonell-Estrany X, Quero-Jiménez J, Fernández-Colomer B, Guzmán-Cabañas J, Echaniz-Urcelay I, et al. Efectividad del palivizumab en la prevención de la infección por virus respiratorio sincitial en prematuros de 32.1 a 35.0 semanas de gestación en España. Acta Pediátrica Española. 2010;**68**:13-18

[70] Resch B, Sommer C, Nuijten MJ, Seidinger S, Walter E, Schoellbauer V, et al. Cost effectiveness of palivizumab for respiratory syncytial virus infection in high-risk children, based on long-term epidemiologic data from Austria. The Pediatric Infectious Disease Journal. 2012;**31**:e1-e8. DOI: 10.1097/INF.0b013e318235455b

Section 3

RSV and Congenital Heart Disease

Chapter 3

Respiratory Syncytial Virus Infections among Children with Congenital Heart Disease

Maja Daurach and Ina Michel-Behnke

Abstract

Infants and children suffering from congenital heart disease represent a patient cohort particularly at risk for severe RSV infections. Most notably the complication rates in lower respiratory tract infections due to RSV among patients with congenital heart disease are significantly higher compared to other patient collectives. Predisposing factors are altered lung mechanics caused by either increased or decreased pulmonary blood flow, both resulting in a ventilation/perfusion mismatch causing decreased pulmonary compliance and higher airway resistance. Randomized controlled trials have shown that immunoprophylaxis with palivizumab is beneficial for CHD patients. Guidelines from different national societies suggest administration of palivizumab for infants with CHD in young age injected monthly throughout the RSV season, if the CHD is considered hemodynamically significant.

Keywords: congenital heart disease (CHD), respiratory syncytial virus (RSV), palivizumab, immunoprophylaxis, lower respiratory tract infection (LRTI), bronchiolitis

1. Introduction

The burden of respiratory syncytial virus (RSV) infections differs markedly between patients. Clinical symptoms might be mild as in a common cold, while at the other end of the spectrum, children suffer from serious complications and negative impact with chronic respiratory problems that can persist into adulthood [1].

Since the 1980s infants and young children with congenital heart defects (CHD) have been shown to be a particularly vulnerable population developing severe lower respiratory tract infections (LRTIs) caused by RSV. The severity of infections in children with CHD was significantly higher than severity in children without CHD [2].

This chapter will provide an overview of the current state of knowledge regarding RSV infections in children with CHD. In particular, we try to elucidate the mechanisms for the susceptibility of children with congenital heart defects to experience critical illness from RSV LRTI.

2. Mechanisms of susceptibility caused by congenital heart disease

In general pulmonary compliance and airway resistance determine the breathing. The airways of young infants have greater airway resistance due to their smaller diameter. Spontaneous breathing of infants is characterized by a functional residual capacity that is less than the closing capacity, which leads to areas of mechanical collapse of the alveoli. As a result the infant itself is more susceptible to develop ventilation/perfusion mismatch and is at higher risk for respiratory problems just from anatomy and pathophysiology irrespective of congenital heart disease [3].

As cardiac and pulmonary function is closely related, the baseline risk of the young infant is increased by several predisposing factors due to CHD.

Pulmonary sequelae and complications of CHD can be anatomical due to compression of the lung by, e.g., cardiomegaly, subsequently causing atelectases or airway malacia. Surgical or anesthesiologic trauma can result in chylothorax, subglottic stenosis, and laryngeal or phrenic nerve palsy leading to respiratory distress [4].

On the other hand, in particular the altered hemodynamics in CHD contributes to an increased vulnerability of the lung. In this context cardiac defects can be categorized in three main categories: (1) those with left-to-right shunt lesions, (2) those with right-to-left shunt lesions, and (3) those with more complex mixing patterns [5].

2.1 Left-to-right shunt lesions: pulmonary overflow

Typically CHDs with left-to-right shunt are acyanotic. They include atrial septal defects (ASDs), ventricular septal defects (VSDs), patent ductus arteriosus (PDA), atrioventricular septal defects (AVSDs), or double outlet right ventricles (DORV) with normally related great vessels (i.e., with VSD physiology). Very rarely coronary fistula or other extracardiac shunts are detected to cause volume overload of the right heart and the lungs.

When there is unrestricted communication between systemic and pulmonary circulation, the shunt volume is depending on the relative resistance in the two circuits with physiologically lower pulmonary resistance. During the normal transition of an infants' blood circulation in the first months of life, the decrease of pulmonary arteriolar resistance leads to an increase of left-to-right shunt. As a result the pulmonary blood flow is increasing (see **Figure 1**). Subsequently the lung volume and pulmonary artery pressure are elevated, and finally the capillary and left atrial pressures increase. At the end lung edema develops with high lung resistance. Alveolar edema and thus higher lung weight result in reduced lung compliance and therefore a decreased ventilation/perfusion ratio leading to intrapulmonary mismatch and eventually hypoxemia.

2.2 Right-to-left shunt lesions: diminished pulmonary flow

Intracardiac right-to-left shunt leads to cyanosis. The basic pathophysiology of the most frequent cyanotic CHD is the tetralogy of Fallot (TOF) and includes an unrestricted communication between systemic and pulmonary circulation (VSD) and obstruction of the pulmonary outlet (see **Figure 2**). In these patients the main hemodynamic difference is reduced pulmonary blood flow, therefore lower lung volume and hypoplastic airways. The hypoplastic airways are more susceptible to obstruction and lead to higher airway resistance. Ventilation/perfusion ratio is increased in these patients causing dead space ventilation, which aggravates an already preexisting hypoxemia.

DOI: http://dx.doi.org/10.5772/intechopen.85552

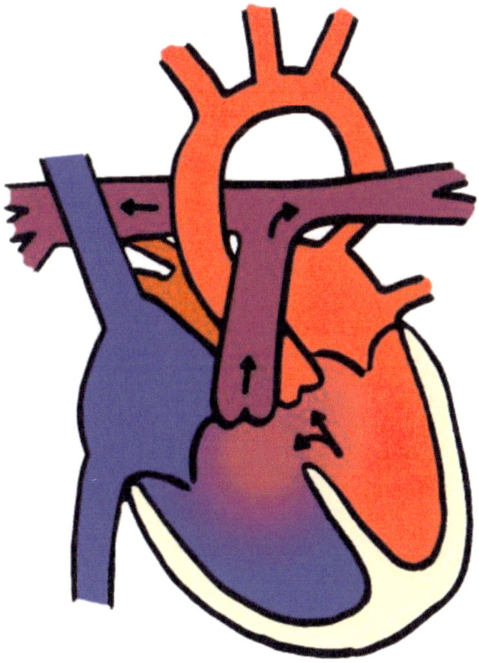

Figure 1.
VSD. Pulmonary overflow due to left-to-right shunt through a ventricular septal defect (VSD).

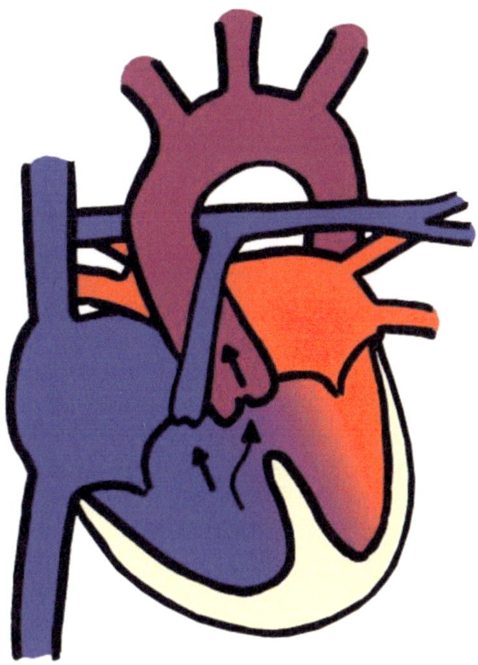

Figure 2.
TOF. Cyanosis due to right-to-left shunt through a VSD when pulmonary stenosis and hypoplastic pulmonary arteries are present in tetralogy of Fallot (TOF).

2.3 Complex CHD with mixed physiology

In patients with complex CHD, cyanosis and relatively increased pulmonary blood flow may occur at the same time. Examples are hypoplastic left heart

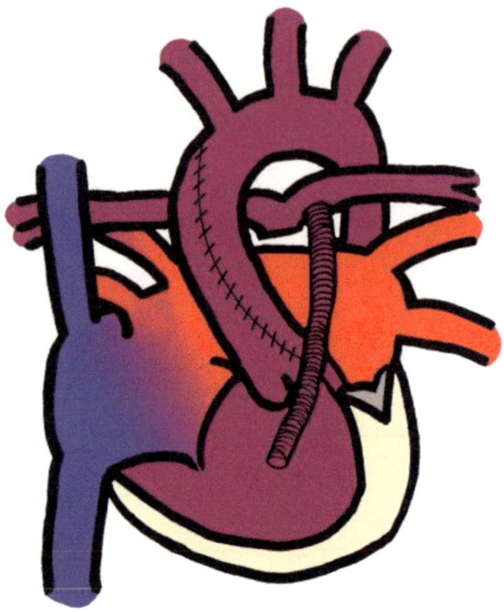

Figure 3.
Norwood-I palliated HLHS. Excessive pulmonary perfusion via Sano shunt leads to relative overflow of the pulmonary arteries, dilated left atrium resulting in higher pulmonary vein pressure causing pulmonary vein congestion.

syndrome (**Figure 3**) or other forms of functionally single ventricle like hypoplastic right heart, tricuspid atresia, or pulmonary atresia. Insertion of systemic to pulmonary shunt as part of the first stage of palliative surgery ideally leads to a balanced pulmonary and systemic perfusion but for the sake of an increased volume load and persisting cyanosis.

These patients are at high risk for ventilation-perfusion mismatch. In addition, impaired ventricular function may contribute to higher pulmonary venous pressures leading to pulmonary venous congestion and subsequently lung edema and higher pulmonary artery pressures [3, 5].

Pulmonary hypertension is known to exacerbate these effects and represents a particular predisposing factor for fatal disease [6].

In the end many complex risk factors are responsible for the susceptibility of young CHD patients. Compromised cardiorespiratory status at baseline, altered pulmonary mechanics, potential cyanosis and/or pulmonary hypertension, and ventilation-perfusion mismatch can increase the negative effects of respiratory disease in this vulnerable patient cohort unable to compensate properly for intercurrent disease. The interplay of the distinct circulation in CHD and the consequences on lung architecture and function contribute to the elevated risk to which these patients are exposed by an RSV infection [5, 7].

3. RSV-related morbidity of children with CHD

RSV accounts for about 20% of all respiratory infections in children below the age of 5 years. Most infections occur in the first 2 years of life. In healthy term infants, hospitalization rates due to RSV LRTI range from 1 to 3%, mainly in the first 6 months of life. Among high-risk populations like preterm infants with or without bronchopulmonary dysplasia (BPD), infants with CHD, Down syndrome, neuromuscular disease, immunosuppressed children, or patients with severe immune deficiency syndromes, hospitalization rates increase up to 10% [8].

As shown in a systematic review as part of the RSV Evidence—A Geographical Archive of Literature (REGAL) series published in 2017 including 38 studies reporting RSV-associated morbidity and mortality, the risk and burden of RSV in CHD still remain serious. RSV hospitalization rates were generally high in young children (<4 years) with CHD varying between 14 and 357/1000 patients. Infants (<2 years) with CHD had a more severe course of RSV infections than patients without CHD. Duration of hospital stay was 4.4–14 days, up to 53% of them requiring intensive care. Case fatality rates of up to 3% were associated with RSV LRTIs in children with CHD. RSV infection in the perioperative period of cardiac surgery and nosocomial infections in ICUs also represent an important cause of morbidity [9].

A recent investigation in Austria analyzed data on RSV-related hospitalizations in infants and small children in their first three RSV seasons (November–April). The study was performed retrospectively and included children with CHD born between 2004 and 2008. The study cohort included 602 patients of whom 451 (74.9%) had hemodynamically not significant CHD (HNS-CHD), 102 (16.9%) had acyanotic, and 49 (8.1%) had cyanotic hemodynamically significant CHD (HS-CHD). Pulmonary hypertension was present in 48 of 151 (31.8%) patients with hemodynamically significant CHD. Overall incidence of RSV-related hospitalizations was 9.6%. Hospitalization rates between hemodynamically significant (10.4%) and not significant CHD (7.3%) did not differ significantly. The median duration of hospitalization was 8.5 days, whereas in HS-CHD the length was 14 days compared to 7 days in HNS-CHD. These results demonstrate the more severe course of RSV infections in children with hemodynamically significant disease. The median duration of supplemental oxygen was 1 day (0–38 days). 22.4% of children were treated at the ICU; the median duration of ICU stay was 10 days (2–70 days), and the median duration of mechanical ventilation was 4 days (0–38 days). Children with hemodynamically significant disease and early heart surgery were less often hospitalized compared to those with delayed cardiac surgery [10].

In order to investigate case fatality rates in young children hospitalized because of RSV LRTIs, a systematic review of 34 articles was conducted in 2012. The case fatality rates for RSV-associated bronchiolitis and pneumonia among patient collectives of children, who are at particular high risk, were compared. The subgroups included (1) preterm infants, born before 37 gestational weeks, (2) children with diagnosed bronchopulmonary dysplasia (BPD) within the first 2 years of life, and (3) children with diagnosed CHD within the first 2 years of life. Case fatality rate among preterm infants was 1.2% (0–8.3%, median 0%), among children with BPD 4.1% (0–10.5%, median 7.0%) and among children with CHD 5.2% (2.0–37%, median 5.9%). While case fatality estimates among children not at high risk ranged from 0 to 1.5% (weighted mean 0.2%, median 0.0%), case fatality rates among children at elevated risk of RSV LRTI were significantly higher with the highest case fatality rate for children with diagnosed CHD [11].

All these papers underline the fact that infants and children with CHD especially when hemodynamically significant represent an extremely sensitive patient collective when it comes to RSV disease. Most strikingly they tend to have a more severe course and worse outcome of LRTIs due to RSV.

4. Prevention of RSV

RSV is the most common cause of LRTIs in infants and toddlers and under certain circumstances like in HS-CHD puts the children at elevated risk to develop respiratory or cardiac failure. Therefore, specific infection control measures are necessary to prevent severe RSV infections [12].

Comprehensive hygiene measures are efficacious and cost-effective in preventing the spread of RSV and should always be advocated as a main prophylactic factor. Breast feeding and avoidance of exposure to tobacco and other smoke are further important facts in the prevention of RSV disease [13, 14]. Delayed day-care attendance in high-risk populations may represent a preventive factor from acquiring RSV infections [15].

As mentioned above early surgical correction of CHD remains a prophylactic factor for severe RSV LRTI [10].

Although vaccine candidates have been in clinical evaluation for nearly 50 years, none, to date, have reached licensing. Palivizumab, a humanized monoclonal antibody, is currently the only intervention licensed for the prevention of severe RSV disease [8].

4.1 Palivizumab prophylaxis

In June 1998, palivizumab was licensed by the US Food and Drug Administration (FDA) for prevention of serious LRTI caused by RSV in pediatric patients, who are at increased risk of severe disease including young children suffering from CHD [16]. The efficacy and safety of palivizumab have been evaluated in many multi-center randomized controlled trials as shown in the following data [17–19].

In 2003 a prospective, randomized, double-blind, placebo-controlled multicenter trial including 1287 children with CHD was published. The study was conducted in the RSV seasons 199–2002 (seventy-six centers in the USA, six in Canada, three in Sweden, four in Germany, six in Poland, four in France, and six in the UK). The primary objective was to compare the safety, tolerance, and efficacy of palivizumab with placebo. The secondary objectives were to determine the effect of monthly administered palivizumab on hospitalization outcomes (total hospitalization duration, days with increased oxygen requirement, incidence, and total days of ICU stays and RSV-associated mechanical ventilation), as well as to describe the effect of cardiac bypass on serum palivizumab levels and determine the palivizumab levels before the second and fifth doses.

Children aged less than 24 months, who had documented hemodynamically significant CHD, not yet corrected or partially corrected, were included. Patients were randomly assigned 1:1 to receive either 5 monthly (every 30 days) intramuscular injections of 15 mg/kg body weight palivizumab or placebo. Children were followed for 150 days for hospitalization and occurrence of adverse events. Monthly prophylaxis with palivizumab was associated with a 45% relative reduction in RSV hospitalization rate (9.7% in the placebo group, 5.3% in the palivizumab group). The length of total hospital stays was reduced by 56% (129 days in the placebo group vs. 57.4 days in the palivizumab group), days with increased oxygen requirement were reduced by 73% (101.5 days placebo vs. 27.9 days palivizumab), days at ICU were reduced by 78%, and days on mechanical ventilation showed a 41% reduction.

Regarding safety and tolerability, the incidence of adverse events in the palivizumab and placebo group was similar. None of the children had drug-related severe adverse events.

The effect of cardiopulmonary bypass on serum palivizumab levels showed a notable decrease (58%) of antibody titers making early restart of palivizumab injections necessary [17].

Another paper documenting the effects of palivizumab in subjects with CHD was published in 2008. During the RSV seasons 2000–2004, data from 19,548 subjects who received immunoprophylaxis with palivizumab were collected prospectively in the palivizumab outcomes registry. One thousand five hundred subjects with CHD (7.7% of the entire cohort) were enrolled. Seventy-one percent had acyanotic CHD. About 1.9% of patients prophylactically treated with palivizumab were hospitalized because of RSV infections, compared to 1.2% of patients included in the registry without CHD, which are low hospitalization rates compared to hospitalization rates before immunoprophylaxis [18].

A further study evaluated the impact of palivizumab prophylaxis on RSV hospitalizations among children with hemodynamically significant CHD by comparing the outcome before and after palivizumab prophylaxis. The American Academy of Pediatrics (AAP) revised the bronchiolitis policy statement and recommended the use of palivizumab in children younger than 24 months old with hemodynamically significant CHD in 2003. California statewide hospital discharge data from years 2000 to 2002 (pre-AAP policy revision) were compared to those from years 2004 to 2006 (post-AAP policy revision). Overall RSV hospitalization rate was 71 per 10,000 children younger than 2 years. 3.0% were children with CHD and 0.50% hemodynamically significant CHD. HS-CHD patients accounted for 0.56% of RSV hospitalizations in 2000–2002, compared to 0.46% RSV hospitalizations in 2004–2006, which means a 19% reduction in RSV hospitalizations among HS-CHD patients after 2003 [19].

4.2 Recommendations for the use of palivizumab in RSV prevention

As shown in many trials, RSV infections still represent increased complication rates in high-risk populations like infants and young children with CHD [2, 10, 11, 20]. There is consensus that palivizumab currently is the only licensed immunoprophylaxis that can and should be offered [21–33].

In this subsection the guidelines and recommendations for palivizumab use in children with CHD in the German-speaking countries will be compared to the guidelines of the USA, the UK, and Canada [21–30].

Table 1 summarizes the most important points of the latest recommendations.

There are substantial differences particularly regarding the age groups of children with CHD, who shall or may receive immunoprophylaxis. All national committees agree on the fact that only children with hemodynamically significant CHD shall get palivizumab. Therefore, if the CHD is considered not hemodynamically significant, i.e., without indication for corrective surgery, intervention or cardiac medication, for example, small atrial septal defects (ASDs), small ventricular septal defects (VSDs), patent ductus arteriosus (PDA), mild aortic or pulmonary stenosis, or mild coarctation, there is no indication for palivizumab. After corrective surgery or intervention is performed, there is no need of palivizumab anymore as the risk is no longer elevated, unless the patients require further cardiac medication or there are other risk factors for severe RSV disease. In this case, the administration of palivizumab after cardiopulmonary bypass shall be given as soon as the patient is stable.

The definition for hemodynamically significant CHD is not consistent throughout the national recommendations.

All of them have in common that cyanotic CHD is considered significant, as well as the presence of pulmonary hypertension. While the recommendations in the USA suggest prophylaxis for moderate and severe pulmonary hypertension (PH), in Switzerland palivizumab shall just be offered for children with severe PH [25, 28].

The latest American Academy of Pediatrics (AAP) recommendations suggest prophylaxis for children, who are born within 12 months of onset of the RSV season and suffer from hemodynamically significant heart disease. Consultation with a cardiologist for decisions about prophylaxis is recommended for patients with cyanotic heart disease. Children with acyanotic HS-CHD, who are receiving medication to control congestive heart failure and will require cardiac surgical procedures, and infants with moderate to severe pulmonary hypertension, as well as children younger than 2 years who undergo cardiac transplantation during the RSV season may be considered for palivizumab prophylaxis [25].

Country	Age	Type of cardiac disease
Austria	<24 m	HS-CHD • Cyanotic or acyanotic • Pulmonary hypertension Myocarditis, dilatative cardiomyopathy, congestive heart failure
	>24 m	High-risk constellation
Germany	<6 m	"Shall" HS-CHD (requires surgery or intervention) • Cyanotic • Pulmonary hypertension • Pulmonary venous congestion Congestive heart failure, requires medication
	6–12 m	"Can"
Switzerland	<12 m	HS-CHD • Cyanotic • Pulmonary hypertension • No surgery before RSV season Congestive heart failure
USA	<12 m	HS-CHD • Cyanotic or acyanotic • Pulmonary hypertension Cardiomyopathy requiring medication for congestive heart failure post-heart
	12–24 m	transplantation
Canada	<12 m	HS-CHD • Cyanotic or acyanotic • Requiring corrective surgery • On cardiac medication
	12–24 m	Ongoing HS-CHD case-by-case
UK	<12 m	HS-CHD Plus significant co-morbidities

Table 1.
Recommendations of different national committees on palivizumab prophylaxis in children with CHD.

The dosage of palivizumab is 15 mg/kg body weight in all recommendations. Prophylaxis shall be provided in the RSV season, which in the northern hemisphere is November until March, with slight differences in some US areas. Five monthly doses of the antibody shall be administered to provide antibody levels for 6 months.

Another important factor is to improve compliance by parental education. A large study from the Canadian registry of palivizumab found out that adherence to the monthly injection regimen was significantly associated with a lower incidence of RSV infections [34].

4.3 Pharmacoeconomics

Due to the high costs of palivizumab, which exceed the costs of RSV-related hospitalizations, the cost-effectiveness of the product is considered controversial [19].

A cost-utility trial performed in Spain published in 2017 estimated the cost-effectiveness of immunoprophylaxis with palivizumab versus placebo among children with CHD. It concluded not only costs of hospitalization but also the impact of delayed cardiac surgery and the complications of performed surgery despite infections. The sequelae of asthma and allergic sensitization were put into calculation as well as indirect costs like parental absence from work. The model demonstrated that palivizumab prophylaxis results in more quality-adjusted life years (QALY) than placebo in children with CHD. Palivizumab prophylaxis was shown to be a cost-effective health-care intervention according to the commonly accepted standards of cost-effectiveness in Spain [35].

A nationwide cost-utility study based on epidemiological data over 16 RSV seasons performed in Austria compared the costs per QALY years in high-risk populations. Overall these long-term epidemiological data suggest that palivizumab is cost-effective in the prevention of RSV diseases in all groups. The results showed lowest costs per QALY years in patients with CHD (8484€) compared to 26,212€ in preterms and 24,654€ in BPD patients [36].

Data on cost-effectiveness still remains controversial but considering the limited treatment strategies for severe RSV infections and possible severe consequences in this especially vulnerable patient cohort may actually justify the costs of this only licensed immunoprophylaxis.

5. Conclusion

LRTIs caused by RSV among children with CHD put patients under high risk of developing respiratory or congestive heart failure. Regarding the increased fatality rates of RSV infections among infants and young children with CHD, immunoprophylaxis with palivizumab may be justified in this patient collective. Used properly (starting in time with regular repetitions throughout the RSV season) palivizumab leads to a significant decrease in RSV-related hospitalization rates, as well as ICU days, days on mechanical ventilation, and days on supplemental oxygen. Unless a vaccine against RSV is found, immunoprophylaxis with palivizumab remains the only way to reduce the burden of RSV disease among this high-risk patient collective at the moment.

Conflict of interest

None.

Author details

Maja Daurach* and Ina Michel-Behnke
Division of Pediatric Cardiology, Department of Pediatrics and Adolescent Medicine, Medical University of Vienna, Vienna, Austria

*Address all correspondence to: maja.daurach@gmail.com

References

[1] Geskey JM, Cyran SE. Managing the Morbidity Associated with Respiratory Viral Infections in Children with Congenital Heart Disease. International Journal of Pediatrics. 2012;**2012**:1-8

[2] MacDonald NE, Hall CB, Suffin SC, Alexson C, Harris PJ, Manning JA. Respiratory Syncytial Viral Infection in Infants with Congenital Heart Disease. New England Journal of Medicine. 1982;**307**(7):397-400

[3] Jung JW. Respiratory syncytial virus infection in children with congenital heart disease: Global data and interim results of Korean RSV-CHD survey. Korean Journal of Pediatrics. 2011;**54**(5):192

[4] Healy F, Hanna BD, Zinman R. Pulmonary Complications of Congenital Heart Disease. Paediatric Respiratory Reviews. 2012;**13**(1):10-15

[5] Cabalka AK. Physiologic risk factors for respiratory viral infections and immunoprophylaxis for respiratory syncytial virus in young children with congenital heart disease. The Pediatric Infectious Disease Journal. 2004;**23**(Supplement):S41-S45

[6] Moler FW, Khan AS, Meliones JN, Custer JR, Palmisano J, Shope TC. Respiratory syncytial virus morbidity and mortality estimates in congenital heart disease patients: a recent experience. Critical Care Medicine. 1992;**20**(10):1406-1413

[7] Resch B, Michel-Behnke I. Respiratory syncytial virus infections in infants and children with congenital heart disease: Update on the evidence of prevention with palivizumab. Current Opinion in Cardiology. 2013;**28**(2):85-91

[8] Resch B. Product review on the monoclonal antibody palivizumab for prevention of respiratory syncytial virus infection. Human Vaccines & Immunotherapeutics. 2017;**13**(9):2138-2149

[9] Checchia PA, Paes B, Bont L, Manzoni P, Simões EAF, Fauroux B, et al. Defining the Risk and Associated Morbidity and Mortality of Severe Respiratory Syncytial Virus Infection Among Infants with Congenital Heart Disease. Infectious Diseases and Therapy. 2017;**6**(1):37-56

[10] Resch B, Kurath-Koller S, Hahn J, Raith W, Köstenberger M, Gamillscheg A. Respiratory syncytial virus-associated hospitalizations over three consecutive seasons in children with congenital heart disease. European Journal of Clinical Microbiology & Infectious Diseases. 2016;**35**(7):1165-1169

[11] Szabo SM, Gooch KL, Bibby MM, Vo PG, Mitchell I, Bradt P, et al. The risk of mortality among young children hospitalized for severe respiratory syncytial virus infection. Paediatric Respiratory Reviews. 2013;**13**:S1-S8

[12] Fixler DE. Respiratory syncytial virus infection in children with congenital heart disease: A review. Pediatric Cardiology. 1996;**17**(3):163-168

[13] Jefferson T, Del Mar CB, Dooley L, Ferroni E, Al-Ansary LA, Bawazeer GA, et al. Physical interventions to interrupt or reduce the spread of respiratory viruses. Cochrane Database of Systematic Reviews. 2011;(7):CD006207

[14] Straňák Z, Saliba E, Kosma P, Posfay-Barbe K, Yunis K, Farstad T, et al. Predictors of RSV LRTI Hospitalization in Infants Born at 33 to 35 Weeks Gestational Age: A Large Multinational Study (PONI). PLoS One. 2016;**11**(6):e0157446

[15] Blanken MO, Korsten K, Achten NB, Tamminga S, Nibbelke EE, Sanders EAM, et al. Population-Attributable Risk of Risk Factors for Recurrent Wheezing in Moderate Preterm Infants During the First Year of Life. Paediatric and Perinatal Epidemiology. 2016;**30**(4):376-385

[16] Simões EAF, Bont L, Manzoni P, Fauroux B, Paes B, Figueras-Aloy J, et al. Past, Present and Future Approaches to the Prevention and Treatment of Respiratory Syncytial Virus Infection in Children. Infectious Diseases and Therapy. 2018;**7**(1):87-120

[17] Feltes TF, Cabalka AK, Meissner HC, Piazza FM, Carlin DA, Top FH, et al. Palivizumab prophylaxis reduces hospitalization due to respiratory syncytial virus in young children with hemodynamically significant congenital heart disease. The Journal of Pediatrics. 2003;**143**(4):532-540

[18] Cohen SA, Zanni R, Cohen A, Harrington M, VanVeldhuisen P, Boron ML, et al. Palivizumab Use in Subjects with Congenital Heart Disease: Results from the 2000-2004 Palivizumab Outcomes Registry. Pediatric Cardiology. 2008;**29**(2):382-387

[19] Chang R-KR, Chen AY. Impact of palivizumab on RSV hospitalizations for children with hemodynamically significant congenital heart disease. Pediatric Cardiology. 2010;**31**(1):90-95

[20] Chiu S-N, Shao P-L, Chen H-C, Lin M-T, Huang L-M, Kao F-Y, et al. Risk of Respiratory Syncytial Virus Infection in Cyanotic Congenital Heart Disease in a Subtropical Area. The Journal of Pediatrics. 2016;**171**:25-30.e1

[21] Pinter M, Geiger R. Empfehlungen zur RSV-Prophylaxe bei Kindern mit angeborenem Herzfehler: Konsensuspapier der Arbeitsgruppe für Kinderkardiologie der österreichischen Gesellschaft für Kinder- und Jugendheilkunde, 2004. Monatsschrift Kinderheilkunde. 2005;**153**(9):878-880

[22] Österreichische Gesellschaft für Kinder- und Jugendheilkunde (ÖGKJ). Konsensuspapier zur Prophylaxe der RSV-Infektion mit Palivizumab und Post-RSV-Atemwegserkrankung. Monatsschrift Kinderheilkunde. 2008;**156**(4):381-383

[23] American Academy of Pediatrics Committee on Infectious Diseases, Committee on Fetus and Newborn. Revised indications for the use of palivizumab and respiratory syncytial virus immune globulin intravenous for the prevention of respiratory syncytial virus infections. Pediatrics. 2003;**112**:1442-1446

[24] Committee on Infectious Diseases. Modified Recommendations for Use of Palivizumab for Prevention of Respiratory Syncytial Virus Infections. Pediatrics. 2009;**124**(6):1694-1701

[25] American Academy of Pediatrics Committee on Infectious Diseases, American Academy of Pediatrics Bronchiolitis Guidelines Committee. Updated guidance for palivizumab prophylaxis among infants and young children at increased risk of hospitalization for respiratory syncytial virus infection. Pediatrics. 2014;**134**(2):e620-e638

[26] The Green Book: Chapter 27a, V2_0. Respiratory syncytial virus immunisation information for public health professionals, including updates; 2015. https://assets.publishing.service.gov.uk/goverPhysical inPhysical Physical ininPhysical innment/uPhysical inploads/system/uploads/attachment_data/file/458469/Green_Book_Chapter_27a_v2_0W.PDF. [accessed 2019-02-15]

[27] Arbeitsgemeinschaft der Wissenschaftlichen Medizinischen Fachgesellschaften. S2k-Leitlinie

"Leitlinie zur Prophylaxe von schweren Erkrankungen durch Respiratory Syncytial Virus (RSV) bei Risikokindern" Aktualisierung 2017/2018. Available from: https://www.awmf.org/uploads/tx_szleitlinien/048-012l_S2k_Prophylaxe-von-schweren_RSV-Erkrankungen-Risikokindern-Palivizumab_2018-11.pdf [Accessed: February 15, 2019]

[28] Agyeman P, Barazzone-Argiroffo C, Hammer J, Heininger U, Nadal D, Pfammatter J-P, et al. Prävention von RSV-Infektionen mit dem humanisierten monoklonalen Antikörper Palivizumab. Swiss Medical Forum – Schweizerisches Medizin-Forum. 2017;**17**(2829):611-614. Available from: https://doi.emh.ch/smf.2017.03033) [Accessed: February 14, 2019]

[29] Preventing hospitalizations for respiratory syncytial virus infection, Position statement of the Canadian pediatric association. 2016. Available from: https://www.cps.ca/en/documents/position/preventing-hospitalizations-for-rsv-infections [Accessed: February 25, 2019]

[30] 2018-2019 Season for Respiratory Syncytial Virus Prophylaxis for High-Risk Infants. 2018. Available from: http://www.health.gov.on.ca/en/pro/programs/drugs/funded_drug/pdf/rsv_info.pdf [Accessed: February 25, 2019]

[31] Bollani L, Baraldi E, Chirico G, Dotta A, Lanari M, Del Vecchio A, et al. Revised recommendations concerning palivizumab prophylaxis for respiratory syncytial virus (RSV). Italian Journal of Pediatrics. 2015;**41**:97

[32] Nakazawa M, Saji T, Ichida F, Oyama K, Harada K, Kusuda S. Guidelines for the use of palivizumab in infants and young children with congenital heart disease. Pediatrics International. 2006;**48**(2):190-193

[33] Chantepie A. bureau de la Filiale de Cardiologie Pédiatrique de la Société Française de Cardiologie. [Use of palivizumab for the prevention of respiratory syncytial virus infections in children with congenital heart disease. Recommendations from the French Paediatric Cardiac Society]. Archives de Pédiatrie. 2004;**11**(11):1402-1405

[34] Chan P, Li A, Paes B, Abraha H, Mitchell I, Lanctôt KL. Adherence to Palivizumab for Respiratory Syncytial Virus Prevention in the Canadian Registry of Palivizumab. The Pediatric Infectious Disease Journal. 2015;**34**(12):e290-e297

[35] Schmidt R, Majer I, García Román N, Rivas Basterra A, Grubb E, Medrano López C. Palivizumab in the prevention of severe respiratory syncytial virus infection in children with congenital heart disease; a novel cost-utility modeling study reflecting evidence-based clinical pathways in Spain. Health Economics Review. 2017;7(1):47. Available from: https://healtheconomicsreview.springeropen.com/articles/10.1186/s13561-017-0181-3) [Accessed: February 8, 2019]

[36] Resch B, Sommer C, Nuijten MJC, Seidinger S, Walter E, Schoellbauer V, et al. Cost-effectiveness of palivizumab for respiratory syncytial virus infection in high-risk children, based on long-term epidemiologic data from Austria. The Pediatric Infectious Disease Journal. 2012;**31**(1):e1-e8

Section 4

RSV Prophylaxis

Chapter 4

RSV: Available Prophylactic Options and Vaccines in Clinical Trials

Debra T. Linfield and Fariba Rezaee

Abstract

Respiratory syncytial virus (RSV) is the leading cause of serious lower respiratory infection (ALRI)-related hospitalization in children worldwide, and a source of morbidity and mortality in high-risk adults. There are strong associations between RSV, persistent wheezing and childhood asthma. Despite extensive research, no effective treatment is available aside from supportive care. The trial of a formalin-inactivated RSV vaccine in the 1960s resulted in priming the severe illness upon natural infection. Palivizumab, a monoclonal antibody approved for RSV prophylaxis in high-risk infants, has only moderately decreased hospital admissions due to RSV infection. Live-attenuated, vector, and protein-based vaccine candidates are being investigated in many clinical trials. Developing a vaccine remains challenging due to finding the right balance between adequate immunogenicity and attenuation of vaccine. Here we review the clinical significance of RSV in infants, young children, high-risk adults, elderly population, pregnant women; clinical manifestations and consequences of RSV infection; the pharmacologic strategies currently available, the current stages of RSV vaccine clinical trials, different strategies, and major hurdles in the development of an effective RSV vaccine.

Keywords: respiratory syncytial virus (RSV), pediatric, respiratory infection, palivizumab, antiviral therapy, immuno-prophylaxis, RSV vaccine, clinical trials

1. Introduction

RSV, a member of the Paramyxoviridae family, is an enveloped, negative-sense, single-stranded RNA virus [1]. Especially within the winter months, it is an important cause of morbidity and mortality among young children, the elderly, and immunocompromised individuals [2]. Infection is transmitted by either direct or indirect contact with respiratory droplets, and prior infection does not result in persistent immunity.

RSV accounts for approximately 2.1 million outpatient visits among children younger than 5 years old [3]. Additionally, there are 177,000 hospitalizations and 14,000 deaths among adults older than 65 years due to RSV infection [4, 5] each year in the United States. Human studies have shown strong associations between RSV, persistent wheezing, and childhood asthma [6–8].

Symptoms usually begin 4–6 days after transmission and present with nasal congestion, rhinorrhea, fever, or cough. RSV is one of the leading causes of lower respiratory tract infection (LRTI), and can cause tachypnea, wheeze, hypoxemia, or respiratory distress, resulting in an emergency department visit or hospital admission [9]. Males are more severely affected than females, and for reasons that are not fully elucidated, Native Americans and Alaskan Native children are more likely than children of other ethnicities to have severe infection requiring hospitalization.

To date, supportive care is the main treatment option for RSV admission [9, 10]. There is no vaccine approved for RSV prophylaxis in the general population. In 1966, the first vaccine for RSV, a formalin-inactivated (FI-RSV) type, was developed. However, it resulted in vaccine-enhanced disease (VED). Among vaccinated infant, 80% developed severe bronchiolitis or pneumonia and two died, compared to only 5% for the placebo group [11]. There was increased eosinophilic and neutrophilic infiltration and mononuclear cells in the lung parenchyma found in the autopsies of two infants that died, which suggests a Th2-biased immune response, however the mechanism of the VED remains unclear [12].

RSV is composed of 10 genes encoding 11 proteins: small hydrophobic (SH) protein, nucleocapsid associated proteins N, P, L, M2–1, and M2–2, the matrix (M) protein, nonstructural proteins NS1 and NS2, glycoprotein (G), and fusion (F) protein. The SH, N, M2–2, NS2, G, and F proteins are the most commonly manipulated proteins in vaccine production (**Figure 1**). The SH protein inhibits cell apoptosis through inhibition of the TNF-α pathway [13]. The N protein initiates encapsidation of the genome, the M2–2 protein mediates the balance between transcription and RNA replication, and the NS2 protein inhibits host interferon (IFN) response [14, 15]. G protein mediates viral attachment to the host cell, while F protein enables fusion of the virus [16, 17]. RSV A and RSV B, the two antigenic subtypes, differ in their amino acid sequence of the G protein and reactivity to antibodies, resulting in differences in disease severity [18]. Targeting the F protein is of particular interest, as it is highly conserved between the two antigenic subgroups.

In this chapter, we will discuss the current and candidate antiviral drugs and prophylactic agents against RSV infection and some of the ongoing clinical trials of RSV vaccines. Evaluation of drugs typically proceeds in a methodical order, from studies in healthy adults, to hospitalized adults, to older seropositive children, to

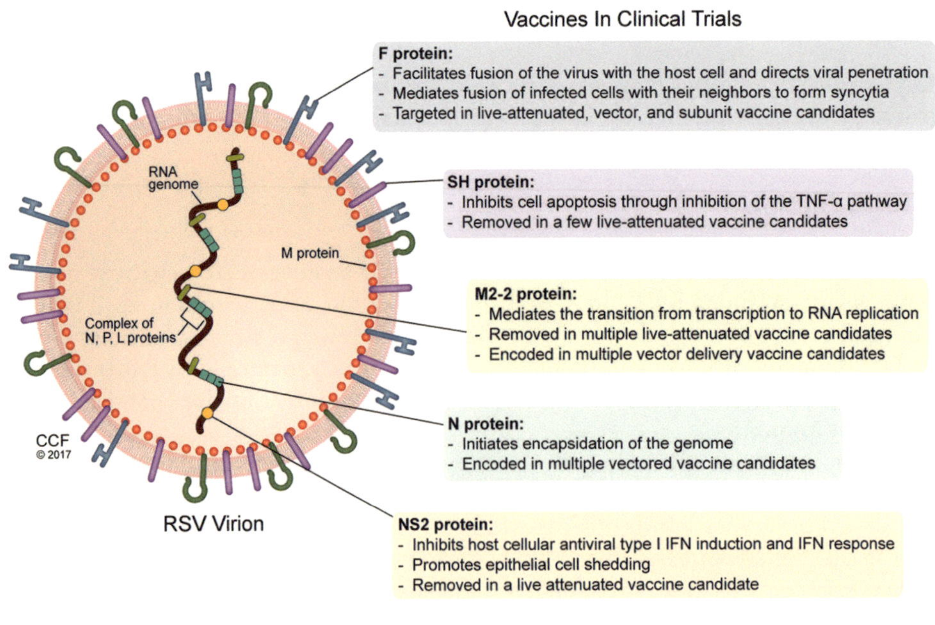

Figure 1.
Current and future options for RSV treatment or prophylaxis. No RSV vaccine is currently on the market, but diverse vaccine candidates, targeting different proteins within the RSV virion, are undergoing clinical trials.

seronegative infants/toddlers. For purposes of this chapter, we will highlight the most recent trials where research is ongoing. We will also elucidate many of the complex hurdles that have impeded progress in the development of an effective vaccine.

2. Available pharmacologic strategies

2.1 Ribavirin

Ribavirin, a synthetic guanosine analogue antiviral agent, was first synthesized in the 1970s. It is believed that ribavirin is phosphorylated intracellularly and can then disrupt purine metabolism by inhibiting inosine monophosphate dehydrogenase, thereby inhibiting nucleic acid synthesis. Furthermore, it promotes antiviral cytokine production and Type 1 T-cell mediated immune responses. Starting in 1993, the American Academy of Pediatrics (AAP) Committee on Infectious Diseases supported the use of Ribavirin for severe RSV infections. However, in 1996, the recommendation changed to "may be considered" [19]. Currently, the use of aerosolized Ribavirin is limited to immunocompromised patients with RSV due to the inconvenient route of delivery, which requires prolonged aerosol administration; risks for potential toxicity, such as teratogenic effects during pregnancy; cost of therapy; and need for hospital admission. The safety of oral ribavirin in moderately to severely immunocompromised adults with PCR-proven RSV infection was examined in a retrospective cohort study. The main outcome of this study was the rate of adverse events, and authors conclude that ribavirin is well tolerated in immunocompromised adults [20]. However, the rate of progression of disease from URTI to the LRTI was not measured. In another retrospective study, immunosuppressed patients were given either oral, intravenous, aerosol or a combination of these treatments and showed that ribavirin therapy reduces progression from RSV URTI to LRTI [21]. In a similar study, Khanna et al. reported that 32% of patients who were treated with ribavirin progressed to LRTI compared to 68% of the untreated group [22]. Their study showed that oral ribavirin therapy was likely as effective as aerosolized therapy. However, because of the sample size and retrospective nature, neither of these studies could determine the precise role of ribavirin therapy in this patient population. In addition, ribavirin is being used for Hepatitis C infection, in conjunction with an interferon agent [23]. Furthermore, a recent study showed that ribavirin inhibited Zika virus replication and Zika virus-induced cell death in mammalian cells [24].

2.2 ALS-008176

ALS-008176, a prodrug of a cytidine nucleoside analogue, decreased viral load and more readily cleared RSV than placebo in a randomized, double-blind clinical trial in healthy adults [25]. However, participants' preexisting immune memory, which may promote RSV clearance, was not assessed [26]. A randomized, double-blind Phase I study assessing both a single and multiple ascending dosing in hospitalized infants (Clinicaltrials.gov identifier #NCT02202356) was completed in February 2018, but results have not been published yet.

2.3 Presatovir

During viral entry, the F protein undergoes conformational changes to fuse with the host cell membrane [17]. Presatovir (GS-5806) is an orally bioavailable agent that inhibits these conformational changes, thereby blocking viral fusion [27]. It was found in a Phase 2a trial with healthy adults (Clinicaltrials.gov identifier

#NCT01756482) to reduce viral load and severity of disease. However, it also caused low neutrophil counts and increased levels of alanine aminotransferase [27]. Despite these adverse events and because of its promise as an efficacious antiviral agent, a Phase 2b, randomized, double-blind trial in RSV-infected hospitalized adults was completed in April 2017 (Clinicaltrials.gov identifier #NCT02135614). The primary outcome was the time-weighted average change in RSV load from baseline to Day 5. There appeared to be no significant differences between Presatovir and placebo (−0.77 vs. −0.89, respectively, p value = 0.46).

3. Currently available and under development immuno-prophylaxis

3.1 RSV-IVIG

RSV Immunoglobulin (RSV-IVIG, RespiGam) is a pooled hyperimmune polyclonal immunoglobulin preparation made from donors with high titers of anti-RSV antibodies. RSV-IVIG significantly reduced morbidity and mortality in high-risk infants [28]. It was initially licensed in 1996, but taken off the market in 2004, due to the need for long intravenous infusion sessions and supervision in a hospital setting, high volume doses resulting in fluid overload in already at-risk infants, and potential risk for blood-borne pathogens [29]. Furthermore, immunizations with live-attenuated viruses, such as the measles/mumps/rubella (MMR) vaccine, need to be postponed until 9 months after RSV-IVIG infusion.

ALX-0171 is an inhaled trivalent nanobody that targets the RSV F protein [30]. A Phase I/IIa in RSV-infected infants and toddlers was recently completed in February 2016 (Clinicaltrials.gov identifier #NCT02309320). A Phase II dose ranging study RSV-infected hospitalized infants was recently completed in May 2018. Results from both studies have not been published yet.

3.2 Palivizumab and motavizumab

Palivizumab (Synagis), developed by MedImmune (Gaithersburg, MD, USA) in 1998, is the only currently approved prophylaxis agent against RSV infection [31]. It has been shown to reduce severe RSV infections by 55% and reduce RSV hospitalizations by 50%. Palivizumab is a humanized monoclonal IgG1 antibody that recognizes the RSV F protein and is administered intramuscularly monthly, for a maximum of 5 months, during the RSV season. It has no significant adverse side effects and other required live-attenuated vaccines can still be administered. However, because of the high cost, it is selectively given to high-risk infants: preterm infants born at <29 weeks of gestation; infants with chronic lung disease (CLD) of prematurity defined as gestational age <32 weeks of gestation and requirement of supplemental oxygen for the first 28 days of life; hemodynamically significant congenital heart disease; and might be considered for neuromuscular disorders that impair the airway clearance [32, 33].

Motavizumab (MEDI-524, Numax), an affinity-matured derivative of palivizumab, was shown to be more efficient than palivizumab with higher virus neutralizing effects [34]. However, it failed to receive FDA approval due to lack of greater clinical efficacy compared to palivizumab and cutaneous hypersensitivity reactions in some treated infants [35].

3.3 Suptavumab

Suptavumab (REGN2222) completed a Phase III trial in July 2017 (Clinicaltrials.gov identifier #NCT02325791). It is a human monoclonal IgG1 antibody against

RSV-F [36]. 1177 preterm infants for whom palivizumab was not recommended were randomly assigned to one of three groups: Group 1 received one dose of intramuscular suptavumab and one dose of placebo, Group 2 received two doses of suptavumab, and Group 3 received two doses of placebo. There were no significant differences between the three groups in terms of the primary outcome of preventing medically attended RSV infection up to Day 150 [36]. All further development of Suptavumab has been stopped.

3.4 MEDI8897

MEDI8897 is another recombinant human monoclonal antibody with a modified Fc region that extends its half-life. MEDI8897 is being developed as RSV prophylaxis for all infants. The phase I (Clinicaltrials.gov identifier #NCT02114268) of study recruited 136 healthy adults, who received either MEDI8897 or placebo intravenously or intramuscularly, a single dose of 300–3000 mg. The half-life of the antibody was 85–117 days across the groups [37]. The phase Ib/IIa of the study, recruited healthy preterm infants with a gestational age of 32–35 weeks. The antibody group received as single intramuscular dose of 10–50 mg MEDI8897. The half-life of the antibody was 62.5–72.9 days. The authors concluded that the antibody has a favorable safety profile and can be administered as single dose during RSV season [38]. A Phase IIb trial in preterm infants' ineligible for Synagis was completed in 2018 and there is a plan for the Phase III trial in healthy full-term and late pre-term infants in 2019.

4. RSV vaccines under development

To date, there is no vaccine against RSV. Developing a vaccine against RSV remains a challenge, as the proper balance is required in eliciting an immune response, while avoiding vaccine-enhanced disease. While many of the proteins within RSV are being manipulated in different vaccine strategies, RSV F comprises a highly conserved amino acid sequence called antigenic site II, between RSV-A and RSV-B antigenic subgroups, and has been considered an important antigen for an RSV vaccine.

Designing a vaccine against RSV requires careful considerations. Infants, the elderly, and pregnant women are the three targeted populations for RSV vaccine development [39]. Each of the three types of vaccines, live-attenuated, vector delivery, and protein based, have benefits and drawbacks that have to be considered when developing vaccine technology (**Table 1**). Live-attenuated vaccines contain extracted components of viral proteins and present antigens most similarly to the naturally occurring infection [40]. They stimulate both humoral and cell-mediated immune responses. Live-attenuated vaccines are employed against many viral diseases, like measles, rubella, polio, rotavirus, varicella, and yellow fever.

Taken from: Rezaee F, Linfield DT, Harford TJ, Piedimonte G. Ongoing developments in RSV prophylaxis: a clinician's analysis. *Curr Opin Virol*. 2017;**24**:70–78.)

One major drawback of live attenuated vaccines is that they cannot be given to patients with compromised immunity including pregnant woman. Vector-delivery system vaccines utilize a non-pathogenic virus genome with inserted portions of RSV proteins. Similar to live-attenuated vaccines, these vaccines increase mucosal IgA and cellular immune responses, yet without the risk of insufficient attenuation [40]. Protein-based vaccines include whole-inactivated viruses, subunit antigens, and particle-based vaccines. Live-attenuated or vector vaccines hold the greatest promise for infants due to the risk of vaccine-enhanced RSV disease. Pregnant women and the elderly are not susceptible to vaccine-enhanced RSV disease, and therefore protein-based RSV vaccines are likely the most effective candidates [40].

	Advantages	Disadvantages
Live-attenuated (For young infants and children <24 months of age)	• Induces immunity • Does not exacerbate future RSV exposure • Administered intranasally	• Need to obtain delicate balance between immunogenicity and adequate attenuation
Vector delivery system (For young infants and children <24 months of age)	• Induced potent cellular and humoral responses in a primate model and preclinical studies • Safer option than live attenuated vaccines in children with no risk of insufficient attenuation	• Prior exposure to the vector and immunological memory against common serotypes may reduce the immune response and limit their use • The potential oncogenicity and pathogenicity of some Adenovirus serotypes
Protein-based (For pregnant women and elderly)	• Maternal immunization could increase transplacental antibody transfer and provide immunity for infants	• High risk of exacerbation for RSV-naïve infants

Table 1.
Advantages and disadvantages of the main strategy categories for RSV vaccine development.

Vaccine type	Current strategies
Live-attenuated	M2–2 gene deletion LID ΔM2–21030s LID cp ΔM2–2 RSV D46/NS2/N/ΔM2–2-HindIII NS2 gene deletion ΔNS2/Δ1313/1314 L RSV 6120/ΔNS2/1030s SH gene deletion MEDI–559 RSV cps2
Vector delivery system	Adenovirus vector GSK3389245A GSK3003891A VXA-RSV-f Ad26.RSV.preF PanAd3-RSV Modified Vaccinia Ankara vector MVA-RSV MVA-BN
Protein-based	Particle based vaccine F-protein nanoparticle Subunit vaccine MEDI-7510

Table 2.
Current vaccine candidates undergoing clinical trials.

Live-attenuated, vector, and protein-based vaccines each possess advantages and disadvantages. Because non-replicating vaccines may elicit enhanced disease in RSV-naïve infants during subsequent infection, replicating or vectored vaccines might be a better choice in this group [41, 42]. Additionally, active immunization for infants is challenging due to passive immunity received from the mother [43]. Because of these factors, different vaccines may be required for different target populations. Understanding these complexities is crucial in RSV vaccine advancement. We will now discuss in depth the different vaccine strategies and current clinical trials in each category. A list of the vaccine candidates is summarized in **Table 2**.

4.1 Live-attenuated vaccines

The tragic results of the formalin-inactivated RSV vaccine in the 1960s spurred research in the development of live-attenuated vaccine candidates. The live virus has parts of the genome deleted and is passaged at gradually lower temperatures. Live-attenuated vaccines require a delicate balance: maintain sufficient viral genome RNA replication to illicit enough antibody response in RSV-naïve infants, yet with a low risk of deattenuation and no harmful effects [44]. Live-attenuated vaccines are, in theory, safe for RSV-naïve infants because it does not exacerbate future exposure to RSV. Furthermore, it may be administered intranasally, which can mimic a milder form of a natural infection, and lead to viral replication in the upper respiratory tract [40]. This will induce mucosal and humoral immunogenicity, despite the potential presence of maternal antibodies acquired transplacentally.

Several live-attenuated RSV vaccine candidates have deletions of a large segment of the M2–2 gene. The M2–2 gene mediates the transition from transcription to RNA replication [14]. *In vitro* studies have shown that M2–2 gene deletion leads to decreased viral RNA replication, but increased F and G protein expression through transcription. This means that the virus is adequately attenuated, yet potentially could lead to augmentation of the neutralizing antibody response [14]. A Phase I study explored the safety of a LID ΔM2–2 vaccine, delivered intranasally to RSV-seronegative infants (aged 6 to 24 months). This vaccine infected the subjects successfully, but the peak shedding titers were higher than wanted, and therefore the study was terminated [45, 46]. Further attenuation to the LID ΔM2–2 vaccine, to counter the high shedding titers, is currently under investigation. The LID ΔM2–21030s vaccine has a mutation conferring temperature sensitivity. A Phase I placebo-controlled study in RSV-seronegative infants aged 6 to 24 months (Clinicaltrials.gov identifier #NCT02794870) completed in July 2017, showed that roughly 60% of vaccine recipients and 27% of placebo recipients had solicited adverse events. Conclusions regarding the LID ΔM2–21030s vaccine have not yet been made. A Phase I LID cp ΔM2–2 vaccine, which in comparison to the LID ΔM2–2 contains 5 amino acid substitutions, was terminated early in seronegative infants 6 to 24 months of age due to indication that the vaccine "did not meet the protocol criteria for a good vaccine candidate" (ClinicalTrials.gov identifier #NCT02890381). We believe that this is because only 6/11 patients in the vaccine arm of the trial were infected with the vaccine virus from Study Day 0–28, thereby suggesting that there was not a strong enough immune response against the vaccine. Another vaccine candidate is RSV D46/NS2/N/ΔM2–2-HindIII that contains one point mutation in the NS2 and N proteins and a modified version of the M2–2 deletion [47]. A Phase I study in RSV-seronegative infants and children 6–24 months of age was completed in May 2018.

Aside from deleting the M2–2 gene, the NS2 gene is another potential "knock-out" gene for a live-attenuated vaccine. The RSV NS2 gene is known to promote epithelial cell shedding and inhibit host IFN response [15]. ΔNS2/Δ1313/1314 L, a vaccine candidate with a deleted NS2 gene, is genetically stable and moderately temperature-sensitive [48]. Another candidate, RSV 6120/ΔNS2/1030s, also has a deleted NS2 gene, in combination with the "1030s" missense mutation, which provides further restriction of replication. Both of these candidates are currently being assessed in both seropositive and seronegative children and infants (Clinicaltrials.gov identifiers #NCT03422237 and #NCT03387137).

Strategies have also targeted the SH gene. The RSV SH gene has multiple functions, including inhibiting cell apoptosis, inhibiting signals from TNF-α, and modifying membrane permeability [49]. One vaccine that has a complete deletion of the SH gene, rA2cp248/404/1030ΔSH, demonstrated restricted antibody response in the subjects, as well as viral genotypic and phenotypic instability primarily due to reversion of the 1030 mutation [42, 48]. MEDI-559 differs from rA2cp248/404/1030ΔSH by silent nucleotide substitutions throughout the viral genome [42, 50]. A Phase I/IIa trial studying the safety and efficacy of MEDI-559, showed a higher incidence of medically attended LRTI in RSV seronegative infants 5 to <24 months of age and in infants 1 to <3 months of age regardless of baseline serostatus within 28 days, as compared to placebo [50]. RSV neutralizing antibodies were detected in 59% of MEDI-559 recipients, in comparison to 9% of placebo subjects. Interestingly, this microneutralization response was lower than the rA2*cp*248/404/1030ΔSH vaccine's response. Adverse events, most notably URTI, occurred in 67% MEDI-559 and 57% placebo recipients, which was not clinically significantly different. Further safety trials are warranted to determine the safety profile of MEDI-559 as there was increased incidence of medically attended LRTI.

In comparison to MEDI-559, RSVcps2 contains 5 nucleotide changes and 1 amino acid substitution. The level of attenuation of RSVcps2 and MEDI-559 was shown to be similar in a study in seronegative chimpanzees [48]. This study also showed that it was temperature-sensitive and phenotypically and genetically stable. A Phase I trial in RSV-seronegative, healthy 6–24 month old children demonstrated that RSVcps2 is safe and effective [51]. Furthermore, unlike MEDI-559, medically attended LRTI was not observed. There were no significant differences in the number of adverse events between the experimental and control groups. However, in comparison to rA2cp248/404/1030ΔSH, RSVcps2 had decreased levels of replication and immunogenicity. The study investigators believe that this is due to the 37 silent nucleotide differences between the two vaccine candidates [51]. An ideal candidate would therefore combine the genetic stability of RSVcps2 and the greater replication and immunogenicity of rA2cp248/404/1030ΔSH. Other ΔSH vaccine candidates include OE4 (RSV-A2-dNS1-dNS2-ΔSH-dGm-Gsnull-line19F) and DB1 (RSV-A2-dNS-ΔSH-BAF), which have both been found to be immunogenic in cotton rats [52, 53].

4.2 Vector delivery systems

Vaccine technology is currently utilizing adenovirus and non-pathogenic viral genomes that can act as immune potentiators of delivery systems. These vaccines contain inserted portions of RSV F, N, and M2–1 proteins [54]. Vector vaccines increase mucosal IgA and cellular immune responses similar to live-attenuated vaccine candidates, yet without the risk of insufficient attenuation [55]. Furthermore, adjuvants used with these vector vaccines could potentially enhance the immune response to the vaccine [56].

GlaxoSmithKline's ChAd155-RSV (GSK3389245A) and GSK3003891A are RSV vaccine candidates encoded by a chimpanzee-derived adenovector. A Phase II trial (Clinicaltrials.gov identifier #NCT02360475) evaluating GSK3003891A in healthy, non-pregnant women aged 18–45 years was recently completed. The study showed that GSK3003891A is both safe and immunogenic. However, a Phase II trial in healthy pregnant women and infants born to vaccinated mothers was canceled due to instability of the PreF antigen during manufacturing. A Phase I study investigating ChAd155-RSV in healthy adults aged 18 to 45 years was recently completed (Clinicaltrials.gov identifier #NCT02491463), and a Phase II study in RSV-seropositive infants aged 12–23 months is underway (Clinicaltrials.gov identifier #NCT02927873). Another adenoviral-vector based RSV vaccine candidate, VXA-RSV-f, expressing the F-protein and a dsRNA adjuvant, is recently completed a Phase I, placebo-controlled, dose-ranging study, using subjects aged 18–49 years. Results have not been released yet.

Adenoviruses of serotype 26 (Ad26) are engineered to comprise a nucleotide sequence encoding RSV F protein, which showed efficacy against RSV in mice and cotton rats [57]. Two Phase I, placebo-controlled studies assessed the administration of Ad26.RSV.FA2, given either once or twice, followed by Ad35.RSV.FA2, and vice versa, to adults aged 18–50 years. Ad26.RSV.FA2 was shown to be safe and well tolerated. There was also increased humoral and cellular immunity for 6 months. Ad26.RSV.preF differs by 5 amino acids and contains the pre-fusion conformation stabilized F protein, and showed increased immunogenicity in comparison to Ad26.RSV.FA2 in pre-clinical studies [58]. It is currently undergoing a Phase II clinical trials in adults aged 18–50 years and RSV-seropositive toddlers aged 12–24 months (Clinicaltrials.gov identifier #NCT03303625) and in healthy adults greater than age 60 (Clinicaltrials.gov identifier #NCT03339713). PanAd3-RSV, a vaccine based on the RSV viral proteins F, N and M2–1 encoded by Simian Adenovirus, completed a Phase I trial in subjects 18–75 years of age (ClinicalTrials.gov identifier #NCT01805921) in 2015, alongside a Modified Vaccinia Virus Ankara (MVA) non-replicating vector vaccine candidate. Both of these vector vaccines contain RSV viral proteins F, N and M2–1.

PanAd3-RSV and MVA-RSV were both safe and effective in cotton rats, mice, and calves [59] and immunogenic in a primate model [54]. Most adverse effects were mild to moderate, self-limiting at the site of injection and the study concluded that the vaccine was safe and immunogenic [60]. Despite the promising results, no current clinical trial is investigating these vaccine candidates. MVA-BN (modified Vaccinia Ankara—Bavarian Nordic) is another MVA-based vaccine undergoing investigation. In August 2018, Bavarian Nordic announced that in a Phase II trial in older adults the MVA-BN vaccine elicited broad antibody and T cell responses to both RSV subtypes that lasted 6 months. Furthermore, a booster shot 1 year later again initiated a robust cellular immune response [61].

4.3 Protein-based vaccines

Pregnant women and the elderly are not susceptible to vaccine-enhanced RSV disease like infants, and therefore RSV protein-based vaccines are most likely the most effective candidates. Protein-based vaccine candidates include whole-inactivated viruses, subunit antigens, and particle-based vaccines. Vaccinating a pregnant woman can provide passive immunity to the fetus, as RSV-neutralizing antibodies have been shown to pass from mother to fetus *in utero* [43]. The higher RSV neutralizing antibody in cord blood was associated with reduced risk of hospitalization and disease severity in RSV infection has been shown by several studies [62, 63]. A recent comprehensive study measured multiple serum neutralizing RSV of the infants presented with primary RSV infection and did not find a direct relationship between the disease severity and level of most of anti–respiratory syncytial virus (RSV) antibody titers. However, they found a significant inverse relationship between antibody titer to RSV F protein and disease severity [64]. This is particularly important as the post-fusion form of RSV F protein has been used in clinical trial [65]. Additionally, experimental studies have shown that RSV infection during pregnancy can alter the offspring's postnatal immunity and airway hyperresponsiveness [66]. Therefore, a protein-based vaccine not only provides immunization for the pregnant woman, but also for the fetus in utero and the offspring once baby is born.

MEDI-7510 is a subunit RSV vaccine candidate that contains the post-fusion F glycoprotein, with or without a glucopyranosyl lipid A (a synthetic TLR-4 agonist) adjuvant [67]. A Phase IIb trial in adults aged 60 and older showed that the vaccine candidate was immunogenic but did not protect the study population from RSV illness [68].

Novavax's RSV F-protein nanoparticle vaccine has been trialed in a few Phase I and II studies in healthy human adults and one study of subjects 24 to <72 months of age, and was found to be well-tolerated and immunogenic in all studies [69, 70].

This vaccine consists of nearly the full-length F glycoprotein. This nanoparticle vaccine prompted transplacental antibody transfer within a guinea pig model [71]. Furthermore, in a Phase II study in healthy women of child-bearing age, the vaccine was well tolerated. The peak of Anti-F IgG antibody was day 14 and persisted for 3 months, optimal for administration during the third trimester [72]. Recently, the immunogenicity, with an aluminum adjuvant, was evaluated in a Phase II trial (Clinicaltrials.gov identifier #NCT02247726) in healthy third-trimester pregnant women. In this study in pregnant women, the primary outcome measures were safety and immunogenicity of the vaccine, as well as its impact on the number of infants with medically-attended RSV LRTI and age of onset of the infection. No results have been posted for this study. However, a Phase III study investigation in the same study population is set to be completed in 2019, thereby suggesting that the Phase II trial met its goals.

5. Conclusions

RSV is one of the most common causes of lower respiratory disease in infants, young children, and the elderly. Treatment is currently limited to supportive care, such as supplemental oxygen, bronchodilators, or corticosteroids. Palivizumab prophylaxis is currently restricted to high-risk infants. There is currently no vaccine to prevent RSV infection. There are many challenges associated with developing an RSV vaccine candidate. When developing a live attenuated vaccine, an equilibrium must be struck between adequate immunogenicity and attenuation of the virus. Non-replicating vaccines, like in some vector-delivery systems and protein-based vaccines, can enhance RSV infection in RSV-naïve infants. Therefore, it may be necessary to develop separate vaccines for each at-risk population: neonates and young children, pregnant women, and the elderly. One highly promising strategy appears to be maternal immunization with a nonreplicating vaccine, as this may provide protection during the first few months of life in the neonate.

Acknowledgements

We thank Dr. Frank Esper (Department of Infectious Disease, Cleveland Clinic Children's) for his insightful comments regarding an earlier version of this chapter. This work was supported by a NIH K08 AI112781 (F.R.) grant.

Conflict of interest

The authors report no conflicts of interest.

Author details

Debra T. Linfield[1] and Fariba Rezaee[2,3]*

1 Cleveland Clinic Lerner College of Medicine of Case Western Reserve University Cleveland, OH, USA

2 Center for Pediatric Pulmonary Medicine, Cleveland Clinic Children's, Cleveland, OH, USA

3 Department of Inflammation and Immunity, Lerner Research Institute Cleveland Clinic Foundation, Cleveland, OH, USA

*Address all correspondence to: rezaeef@ccf.org

References

[1] Wright M, Piedimonte G. Respiratory syncytial virus prevention and therapy: Past, present, and future. Pediatric Pulmonology. 2011;**46**(4):324-347

[2] Geoghegan S et al. Mortality due to respiratory syncytial virus. Burden and risk factors. American Journal of Respiratory and Critical Care Medicine. 2017;**195**(1):96-103

[3] Hall CB et al. The burden of respiratory syncytial virus infection in young children. The New England Journal of Medicine. 2009;**360**(6):588-598

[4] Falsey AR et al. Respiratory syncytial virus infection in elderly and high-risk adults. The New England Journal of Medicine. 2005;**352**(17):1749-1759

[5] McClure DL et al. Seasonal incidence of medically attended respiratory syncytial virus infection in a community cohort of adults >/=50 years old. PLoS One. 2014;**9**(7):e102586

[6] Stein RT et al. Respiratory syncytial virus in early life and risk of wheeze and allergy by age 13 years. Lancet. 1999;**354**(9178):541-545

[7] Stensballe LG et al. The causal direction in the association between respiratory syncytial virus hospitalization and asthma. The Journal of Allergy and Clinical Immunology. 2009;**123**(1):131-137. e1

[8] Thomsen SF et al. Exploring the association between severe respiratory syncytial virus infection and asthma: A registry-based twin study. American Journal of Respiratory and Critical Care Medicine. 2009;**179**(12): 1091-1097

[9] Piedimonte G. RSV infections: State of the art. Cleveland Clinic Journal of Medicine. 2015;**82**(11 Suppl 1):S13-S18

[10] Rezaee F et al. Ongoing developments in RSV prophylaxis: A clinician's analysis. Current Opinion in Virology. 2017;**24**:70-78

[11] Acosta PL, Caballero MT, Polack FP. Brief history and characterization of enhanced respiratory syncytial virus disease. Clinical and Vaccine Immunology. 2015;**23**(3):189-195

[12] Knudson CJ et al. RSV vaccine-enhanced disease is orchestrated by the combined actions of distinct CD4 T cell subsets. PLoS Pathogens. 2015;**11**(3):e1004757

[13] Fuentes S et al. Function of the respiratory syncytial virus small hydrophobic protein. Journal of Virology. 2007;**81**(15):8361-8366

[14] Bermingham A, Collins PL. The M2-2 protein of human respiratory syncytial virus is a regulatory factor involved in the balance between RNA replication and transcription. Proceedings of the National Academy of Sciences of the United States of America. 1999;**96**(20): 11259-11264

[15] Liesman RM et al. RSV-encoded NS2 promotes epithelial cell shedding and distal airway obstruction. The Journal of Clinical Investigation. 2014;**124**(5):2219-2233

[16] Techaarpornkul S, Barretto N, Peeples ME. Functional analysis of recombinant respiratory syncytial virus deletion mutants lacking the small hydrophobic and/or attachment glycoprotein gene. Journal of Virology. 2001;**75**(15):6825-6834

[17] Krarup A et al. A highly stable prefusion RSV F vaccine derived from structural analysis of the fusion mechanism. Nature Communications. 2015;**6**:8143

[18] Gilca R et al. Distribution and clinical impact of human respiratory syncytial virus genotypes in hospitalized children over 2 winter seasons. The Journal of Infectious Diseases. 2006;**193**(1):54-58

[19] American Academy of Pediatrics Committee on Infectious Diseases. Use of ribavirin in the treatment of respiratory syncytial virus infection. Pediatrics. 1993;**92**(3):501-504

[20] Marcelin JR et al. Oral ribavirin therapy for respiratory syncytial virus infections in moderately to severely immunocompromised patients. Transplant Infectious Disease. 2014;**16**(2):242-250

[21] Avetisyan G et al. Respiratory syncytial virus infection in recipients of allogeneic stem-cell transplantation: A retrospective study of the incidence, clinical features, and outcome. Transplantation. 2009; **88**(10):1222-1226

[22] Khanna N et al. Respiratory syncytial virus infection in patients with hematological diseases: Single-center study and review of the literature. Clinical Infectious Diseases. 2008;**46**(3):402-412

[23] Novembrino C et al. Interferon-ribavirin therapy induces serum antibodies determining 'rods and rings' pattern in hepatitis C patients. Journal of Viral Hepatitis. 2014;**21**(12): 944-949

[24] Kamiyama N et al. Ribavirin inhibits Zika virus (ZIKV) replication in vitro and suppresses viremia in ZIKV-infected STAT1-deficient mice. Antiviral Research. 2017;**146**:1-11

[25] DeVincenzo JP et al. Activity of oral ALS-008176 in a respiratory syncytial virus challenge study. The New England Journal of Medicine. 2015;**373**(21):2048-2058

[26] Arasaratnam R. ALS-008176 for respiratory syncytial virus infection. The New England Journal of Medicine. 2016;**374**(14):1391

[27] German P et al. Phase 1 first-in-human, single- and multiple-ascending dose, and food effect studies to assess the safety, tolerability, and pharmacokinetics of presatovir for the treatment of respiratory syncytial virus infection. Journal of Clinical Pharmacology. 2018;**58**(8):1025-1034

[28] The PREVENT Study Group. Reduction of respiratory syncytial virus hospitalization among premature infants and infants with bronchopulmonary dysplasia using respiratory syncytial virus immune globulin prophylaxis. Pediatrics. 1997;**99**(1):93-99

[29] Roymans D, Koul A. Treatment of respiratory syncytial virus infection: Past, present and future. In: Resch B, editor. Human Respiratory Syncytial Virus Infection. London, United Kingdom: InTech; 2011

[30] Larios Mora A et al. Delivery of ALX-0171 by inhalation greatly reduces respiratory syncytial virus disease in newborn lambs. MAbs. 2018;**10**(5):778-795

[31] The IMpact-RSV Study Group. Palivizumab, a humanized respiratory syncytial virus monoclonal antibody, reduces hospitalization from respiratory syncytial virus infection in high-risk infants. Pediatrics. 1998; **102**(3 Pt 1):531-537

[32] American Academy of Pediatrics Committee on Infectious, D. and C. American Academy of Pediatrics Bronchiolitis Guidelines. Updated guidance for palivizumab prophylaxis among infants and young children at increased risk of hospitalization for respiratory syncytial virus infection. Pediatrics. 2014;**134**(2):415-420

[33] Meissner HC. More on viral bronchiolitis in children. The New England Journal of Medicine. 2016;**375**(12):1200

[34] Weisman LE. Motavizumab, a second-generation humanized mAb for the prevention of respiratory syncytial virus infection in high-risk populations. Current Opinion in Molecular Therapeutics. 2009;**11**(2):208-218

[35] O'Brien KL et al. Efficacy of motavizumab for the prevention of respiratory syncytial virus disease in healthy Native American infants: A phase 3 randomised double-blind placebo-controlled trial. The Lancet Infectious Diseases. 2015;**15**(12):1398-1408

[36] Tripp RA et al. Respiratory syncytial virus: Targeting the G protein provides a new approach for an old problem. Journal of Virology. 2018;**92**(3):e01302-e01317

[37] Griffin MP et al. Safety, tolerability, and pharmacokinetics of MEDI8897, the respiratory syncytial virus prefusion F-targeting monoclonal antibody with an extended half-life, in healthy adults. Antimicrobial Agents and Chemotherapy. 2017;**61**(3):e01714-e01716

[38] Domachowske JB et al. Safety, tolerability and pharmacokinetics of MEDI8897, an extended half-life single-dose respiratory syncytial virus prefusion F-targeting monoclonal antibody administered as a single dose to healthy preterm infants. The Pediatric Infectious Disease Journal. 2018;**37**(9):886-892

[39] Graham BS. Vaccine development for respiratory syncytial virus. Current Opinion in Virology. 2017;**23**:107-112

[40] Karron RA, Buchholz UJ, Collins PL. Live-attenuated respiratory syncytial virus vaccines. Current Topics in Microbiology and Immunology. 2013;**372**:259-284

[41] Wright PF et al. The absence of enhanced disease with wild type respiratory syncytial virus infection occurring after receipt of live, attenuated, respiratory syncytial virus vaccines. Vaccine. 2007;**25**(42):7372-7378

[42] Karron RA et al. Identification of a recombinant live attenuated respiratory syncytial virus vaccine candidate that is highly attenuated in infants. The Journal of Infectious Diseases. 2005;**191**(7):1093-1104

[43] Chu HY et al. Respiratory syncytial virus transplacental antibody transfer and kinetics in mother-infant pairs in Bangladesh. The Journal of Infectious Diseases. 2014;**210**(10):1582-1589

[44] Le Nouen C et al. Genetic stability of genome-scale deoptimized RNA virus vaccine candidates under selective pressure. Proceedings of the National Academy of Sciences of the United States of America. 2017;**114**(3):E386-E395

[45] McFarland E. Phase I Placebo Controlled Study of the Infectivity, Safety and Immunogenicity of a Single Dose of a Recombinant Live-Attenuated Respiratory Syncytial Virus Vaccine, LID ΔM2-2 1030s, Lot RSV#010A, Delivered as Nose Drops to RSV-Seronegative Infants 6 to 24 Months of Age. National Institutes of Health (NIH), Washington: DC IMPAACT Network; 2016. pp. 16-20

[46] McFarland E et al. High infectivity of recombinant live-attenuated respiratory syncytial virus vaccine (RSV LID ΔM2-2) in infants and children. Open Forum Infectious Diseases. 2015;**2**:1924

[47] McFarland E. Phase I Placebo-Controlled Study of the Infectivity, Safety and Immunogenicity of a Single

Dose of a Recombinant Live-Attenuated Respiratory Syncytial Virus Vaccine, D46/NS2/N/ΔM2-2-HindIII, Lot RSV#011B, Delivered as Nose Drops to RSV-Seronegative Infants 6 to 24 Months of Age. National Institute of Allergy and Infectious Diseases, Washington, DC: IMPAACT Network; 2017

[48] Luongo C et al. Respiratory syncytial virus modified by deletions of the NS2 gene and amino acid S1313 of the L polymerase protein is a temperature-sensitive, live-attenuated vaccine candidate that is phenotypically stable at physiological temperature. Journal of Virology. 2013;**87**(4):1985-1996

[49] Collins PL, Fearns R, Graham BS. Respiratory syncytial virus: Virology, reverse genetics, and pathogenesis of disease. Current Topics in Microbiology and Immunology. 2013;**372**:3-38

[50] Malkin E et al. Safety and immunogenicity of a live attenuated RSV vaccine in healthy RSV-seronegative children 5 to 24 months of age. PLoS One. 2013;**8**(10):e77104

[51] Buchholz UJ et al. Live respiratory syncytial virus (RSV) vaccine candidate containing stabilized temperature-sensitivity mutations is highly attenuated in rsv-seronegative infants and children. The Journal of Infectious Diseases. 2018;**217**(9):1338-1346

[52] Rostad CA et al. A recombinant respiratory syncytial virus vaccine candidate attenuated by a low-fusion F protein is immunogenic and protective against challenge in cotton rats. Journal of Virology. 2016;**90**(16):7508-7518

[53] Stobart CC et al. A live RSV vaccine with engineered thermostability is immunogenic in cotton rats despite high attenuation. Nature Communications. 2016;**7**:13916

[54] Pierantoni A et al. Mucosal delivery of a vectored RSV vaccine is safe and elicits protective immunity in rodents and nonhuman primates. Molecular Therapy - Methods & Clinical Development. 2015;**2**:15018

[55] Anderson LJ et al. Strategic priorities for respiratory syncytial virus (RSV) vaccine development. Vaccine. 2013;**31**(Suppl 2):B209-B215

[56] Jorquera PA, Tripp RA. Synthetic biodegradable microparticle and nanoparticle vaccines against the respiratory syncytial virus. Vaccine. 2016;**4**(4):E45

[57] Widjojoatmodjo MN et al. Recombinant low-seroprevalent adenoviral vectors Ad26 and Ad35 expressing the respiratory syncytial virus (RSV) fusion protein induce protective immunity against RSV infection in cotton rats. Vaccine. 2015;**33**(41):5406-5414

[58] Polack FP. Update on RSV Vaccine Development. Fundacion. Geneva, Switzerland: INFANT; 2017

[59] Green CA et al. Safety and immunogenicity of novel respiratory syncytial virus (RSV) vaccines based on the RSV viral proteins F, N and M2-1 encoded by simian adenovirus (PanAd3-RSV) and MVA (MVA-RSV); protocol for an open-label, dose-escalation, single-centre, phase 1 clinical trial in healthy adults. BMJ Open. 2015;**5**(10):e008748

[60] Green CA et al. Chimpanzee adenovirus- and MVA-vectored respiratory syncytial virus vaccine is safe and immunogenic in adults. Science Translational Medicine. 2015;**7**(300):300ra126

[61] Bavarian Nordic Announces Positive Data from Phase 2 Extension Study of its Universal RSV Vaccine. 2018, GlobeNewsWire: Copenhagen, Denmark

[62] Stensballe LG et al. Respiratory syncytial virus neutralizing antibodies in cord blood, respiratory syncytial virus hospitalization, and recurrent wheeze. The Journal of Allergy and Clinical Immunology. 2009;**123**(2):398-403

[63] Glezen WP et al. Risk of respiratory syncytial virus infection for infants from low-income families in relationship to age, sex, ethnic group, and maternal antibody level. The Journal of Pediatrics. 1981;**98**(5):708-715

[64] Walsh EE et al. Virus-specific antibody, viral load, and disease severity in respiratory syncytial virus infection. The Journal of Infectious Diseases. 2018;**218**(2):208-217

[65] Rossey I et al. Clinical potential of prefusion RSV F-specific antibodies. Trends in Microbiology. 2018;**26**(3):209-219

[66] Brown PM et al. Prenatal exposure to respiratory syncytial virus alters postnatal immunity and airway smooth muscle contractility during early-life reinfections. PLoS One. 2017;**12**(2):e0168786

[67] Broadbent L et al. Respiratory syncytial virus, an ongoing medical dilemma: An expert commentary on respiratory syncytial virus prophylactic and therapeutic pharmaceuticals currently in clinical trials. Influenza and Other Respiratory Viruses. 2015;**9**(4):169-178

[68] Falloon J et al. An adjuvanted, postfusion F protein-based vaccine did not prevent respiratory syncytial virus illness in older adults. The Journal of Infectious Diseases. 2017; **216**:1362-1370

[69] Glenn GM et al. A randomized, blinded, controlled, dose-ranging study of a respiratory syncytial virus recombinant fusion (F) nanoparticle vaccine in healthy women of childbearing age. The Journal of Infectious Diseases. 2016;**213**(3):411-422

[70] Glenn GM et al. Safety and immunogenicity of a Sf9 insect cell-derived respiratory syncytial virus fusion protein nanoparticle vaccine. Vaccine. 2013;**31**(3):524-532

[71] Glenn GM et al. Modeling maternal fetal RSV F vaccine induced antibody transfer in guinea pigs. Vaccine. 2015;**33**(47):6488-6492

[72] August A et al. A Phase 2 randomized, observer-blind, placebo-controlled, dose-ranging trial of aluminum-adjuvanted respiratory syncytial virus F particle vaccine formulations in healthy women of childbearing age. Vaccine. 2017;**35**(30):3749-3759

Chapter 5

Hurdles in Vaccine Development against Respiratory Syncytial Virus

Muhammad Shafique, Muhammad Asif Zahoor, Muhammad Imran Arshad, Bilal Aslam, Abu Baker Siddique, Muhammad Hidayat Rasool, Muhammad Usman Qamar and Muhammad Usman

Abstract

Respiratory syncytial virus (RSV) infection is a major cause of severe respiratory disease in infants and young children worldwide and also forms a serious threat for the elderly. Vaccination could significantly relieve the burden of the RSV disease. However, unfortunately there is no licensed vaccine available so far. This is partly due to disastrous outcome of a clinical trial of formalin-inactivated RSV (FI-RSV) in children in 1960s; leading to enhanced respiratory disease upon natural infection. These findings contributed significantly to the delay of RSV vaccine development. Other key obstacles in development of RSV vaccine such as a peak of severe disease at 2–3 months of age, challenging biochemical behavior of key vaccine antigens and dependence on animal models that may not truly reflect human disease processes. These challenges could be overcome through maternal immunization, structure-based engineering of vaccine antigens, the design of a novel platform for safe infant immunization, and the development of improved animal models. Currently, several vaccine candidates are in pre-clinical and clinical trials targeting the diverse age groups; young children or older adults from the infection or can reduce incidence, mortality and morbidity among the RSV infected individuals.

Keywords: respiratory syncytial virus, vaccines, adaptive immune response, adjuvants, animal models, infants, elderly, enhanced respiratory disease, innate immune response

1. Introduction

Respiratory syncytial virus (RSV) infection is a major cause of lower respiratory tract diseases among infants, young children and immune-compromised individuals. RSV infection provides partial immunity and reinfection may occur often throughout life. Therefore, RSV infection forms a severe threat in chronically ill adults and the elderly [1]. Current studies have demonstrated that RSV also a main cause of mortality among the elderly, indeed to similar extents as does influenza [2]. Presently, the only approved medication against RSV infection is a prophylactic monoclonal antibody, i.e., Palivizumab, which is given as a prophylaxis to high-risk

IntechOpen

Target groups	Considerations	Vaccines approaches
Infants (<6 months)	**Goal:** Prevent severe complications **Challenges:** Less developed immune system; more susceptible to disease; FI-RSV enhanced respiratory disease history, maternal Abs present	1. Live-attenuated vaccines 2. Gene based vectors 3. Virus chimeric vectors
Children (6–24 months old)	**Goal:** Prevent severe complications **Challenges:** To achieve the clinical end point is not easy; FI-RSV enhanced respiratory disease history	4. Gene based vectors 5. Live-attenuated vaccines 6. Virus chimeric vectors
Elderly people (>65 years)	**Goal:** Po provide protection from infections and complications **Challenges:** Lot of previous infections can decrease response to vaccine; necessary to boost up protection provided by natural infection; absence of indicators for severity of disease, diagnosis difficult	7. Subunit proteins having adjuvant 8. Gene based vectors having subunit proteins 9. Vaccines including virus like particles with adjuvants
Pregnant women	**Goal:** To prevent transmission from mother to infants, maximize the protection of infants **Challenges:** Lot of previous infections can decrease response to vaccine, necessary to boost up the antibody level for protection of infants	10. Subunit proteins in combination with standard adjuvants 11. Vaccines having virus like particles with adjuvants

Table 1.
Key target groups for vaccine candidates.

infants [3]. Despite the isolation and characterization of the virus in 1956, efforts to develop a safe vaccine have been unsuccessful so far. In a clinical trial conducted in young children in the 1960s, a formalin-inactivated RSV (FI-RSV) vaccine did not protect against infection rather led to enhanced respiratory disease (ERD) upon subsequent exposure of the vaccinees to the natural virus. These findings that inactivated RSV vaccines may prime for ERD has contributed significantly to the delay of vaccine development. Other major challenges for development of RSV vaccine are a disease severity at 2–3 months of age, challenging biochemical behavior of key vaccine antigens and dependence on animal models that may not exactly mimic human disease processes. These challenges could be overcome through maternal immunization, structure-based engineering of vaccine antigens, the design of a novel strategy for safe immunization of infants, and the development of better animal models (**Table 1**).

2. Respiratory syncytial virus

RSV is an enveloped non-segmented negative-sense single-stranded (ss) RNA virus belonging to the *Orthopneumovirus* genus and *Pneumoviridae* family [4]. Two serotypes of RSV have been recognized i.e., RSV A and RSV B [4].

The RSV genome comprises 10 genes of 15.2 kb nucleotides encodes 11 proteins [5]. RSV comprises of a nucleocapsid enclosed by a lipid envelope with a diameter of 150–300 nm (**Figure 1**: RSV particle and RSV-genome). RSV expresses two non-structural proteins such as NS1 and NS2. These are detected only in RSV-infected cells and are not packaged into the virion. They mainly serve to inhibit type I interferon responses [7]. Eight RSV proteins are present in the virion particles. Among these structural proteins, three are membrane proteins: the attachment protein G, the fusion protein F and the small hydrophobic protein (SH). The heavily

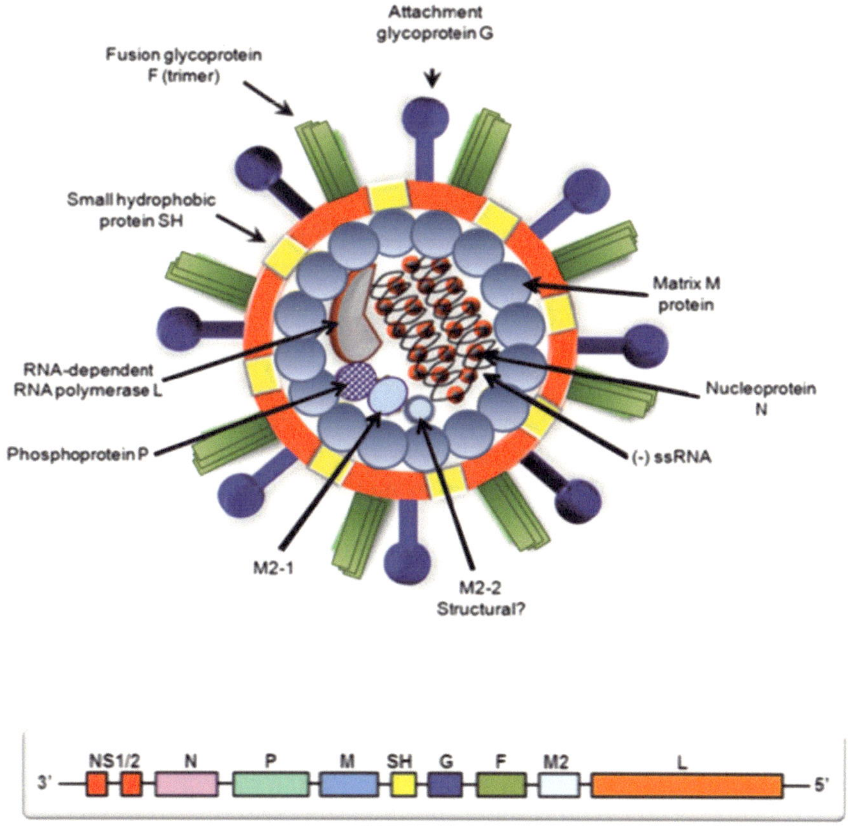

Figure 1.
Schematic representation of the RSV virion and its genome composition (adapted and modified with permission from [6]).

glycosylated G protein is responsible for viral attachment to the cell. The F protein not only contributes to binding of the virus to cells, but also plays a crucial part during entry of virus by mediating fusion of the viral envelope with the cell membrane, thereby allowing deposition of the viral genome into the cytosol [8]. Besides this, F protein is a mediator of syncytium formation [5]. The function of the SH protein, which is mostly found in the infected-cell membrane, is unknown [9]. Other viral structural proteins are the nucleocapsid protein (N), the matrix protein (M), the phosphoprotein (P), the RNA-dependent RNA polymerase (L) and the M2 gene product M2-1: all these proteins are located inside the viral particle. Whereas the M2-2 gene product is packaged in the virion is currently unknown [10]. The function of the matrix (M) protein is to connect the viral nucleocapsid with the lipid envelops and it is also responsible for viral particle assembly. The M2-2 protein is involved in regulation of viral transcription [11]. M2-1 functions as transcription-elongation factor [12]. The phosphoprotein (P) and nucleocapsid protein (N) are essential for transcriptional activity, while the L protein has RNA polymerase activity.

3. Epidemiology

RSV infections have a distribution worldwide. These infections are more common during the winter season in temperate climates. However, RSV infections may occur throughout the year in tropical climates, but can be more frequent in the monsoon season in some areas [13–15]. Although infection can be established in several laboratory animals, however, natural infection with RSV appears to be limited to apes and humans [16]. RSV transmission occurs via direct contact or contact with contaminated surfaces that harbor respiratory secretions. The virus can survive for many hours on toys or other substances, which explains the high rate of nosocomial RSV infections particularly in pediatric wards. The incubation period for RSV infection ranges between 2 and 7 days [17]. Almost 70% of newborns are infected in the first year of their life. By the age of 2 years, almost all children have been infected and over 50% will have been infected twice [18]. RSV infections are common in the population and re-infections probably occur frequently. In a study conducted by Hall et al., 1991, almost 25% of adult volunteers could be re-infected with RSV of the same group, 2 months after a natural infection [19].

RSV infection is the major source of severe respiratory illness in infants and young children and is the most frequent cause of hospitalization of infants and young children in industrialized countries [20]. RSV infections differ in disease severity, from a mild cold to bronchiolitis or pneumonia. Almost 3% of infants infected with RSV need hospitalization due to respiratory failure and feeding problems [21]. Among the hospitalized infants, 20% need mechanical ventilation [22]. The highest morbidity of RSV disease is seen in children under the age of 6 months [23] and in children with associated risk factors such as prematurity, broncho-pulmonary dysplasia, congenital heart disease with increased pulmonary circulation or immune deficiency [24–27]. According to WHO estimates, RSV disease burden is ~64 million cases and 160,000 deaths per year worldwide. In USA, about 85,000–144,000 infants are admitted to hospitals with RSV infection annually which corresponds to 20–25% of pneumonia cases and about 70% bronchiolitis cases in the hospital [28, 29]. The elderly people are also at risk for extreme RSV disease and almost 14,000–62,000 RSV-associated hospitalizations of the elderly occur in USA with an approximate annual cost of RSV pneumonia-related hospitalizations of $150–680 million [30, 31].

4. Pathogenesis

After RSV infection, virus primarily multiplies in the epithelial cells of the nasopharynx [32]. The exact mechanism by which RSV spreads to the lower respiratory tract is not clear yet. Currently, it is not known why the disease progression is mild in most children, but severe in a small subgroup. Different studies have described associations between disease severity and genes involved in allergic responses, like IL-4 and IL-4 receptor genes, and genes for inflammatory cytokines, e.g., IL-6 and IL-8 [33]. Furthermore, up-regulation of chemokines during RSV infection is associated with disease severity. For example, CCL11 (eotaxin), RANTES (CCL5) and MIP1α have been found in higher levels in cases with more severe RSV infection and ERD [34, 35].

Several other factors could be associated with disease severity, for example, environmental factors, patient intrinsic factors, virus strain and viral load. Environmental factors like a high number of siblings, attendance of day-care centers and socio-economic status can enhance the chance of early exposure and may increase the risk of developing lower respiratory tract disease [36]. Other factors like geographical area, parental smoking and the use of wood-burning stoves have also been linked to an enhanced risk of severe RSV infections [37–40]. Patient-intrinsic factors like a compromised respiratory function, e.g., bronchopulmonary dysplasia (BPD) [25], or congenital heart disease with increased pulmonary circulation may significantly enhance the risk to develop severe RSV infection [41]. It is reported in some studies that RSV-strain A is responsible for more severe disease [42], while other studies report no difference between RSV A and B strains [43, 44]. Furthermore, the course of lower respiratory disease was found to be associated with a high viral load [45]. Finally, RSV-specific immunity induced by vaccination may also be involved in immunopathological mechanisms leading to enhanced disease. This hypothesis is mainly based on experimental animal data [46], and on observations from a clinical trial where, as indicated above, infants were vaccinated with FI-RSV vaccine, which resulted in enhanced respiratory disease (ERD) upon natural infection [47–49]. The notion that inactivated-RSV preparations can prime for ERD is one of the factors that has delayed the development of an effective RSV vaccine.

5. Therapeutic approaches against RSV

Only supportive treatment is available. In supportive treatment we can use corticosteroids, bronchodilator and oxygen supplement. These are effective to some extent [50]. It is viral infection, so the use of antibiotics is not recommended, but according to some studies antibiotics can be used to some extent but not regularly to prevent the secondary bacterial infection such as urinary tract infections [51]. Corticosteroids also cannot be used routinely because they are the immunosuppressors [52]. The only recommended antiviral RSV treatment at clinical level is ribavirin. Studies are present which indicate the conflicting results of ribavirin use. It is also less effective and very costly. Due to the conflicting results of ribavirin, American Academy of Science recommendation is that ribavirin should not be routinely used in children having the symptoms of bronchiolitis [53]. Ribavirin completes its function by preventing the polymerase of virus. So ribavirin can inhibit both the DNA and RNA viruses. Ribavirin action may result in anemia and other adverse reactions such as hypersensitivity. According to few studies, ophthalmologic disorders also have been noted after the use of ribavirin. All these side-effects lead towards the limited use of ribavirin in RSV treatment [54]. A study indicated that ribavirin might be used in target groups such as children having RSV infection with comorbid immunosuppression, but it is necessary to investigate and verify more data about its recommendation [55, 56]. It has also been noted that once the disease has occurred, no effective treatment is available for preventing the disease. Another study explained its failure in treatment describing that inhibiting the replication of virus alone is not enough to block the virus mediated pathogenesis in host. So, due to limited treatment options and high disease burden, it is necessary to discover the new treatment as well as prophylactic policies.

Now there is focus on F protein for the development of anti-RSV drugs as well as vaccines. Researches are being conducted for the development of numerous antiviral drugs and antibodies that are in preclinical development stage. Some of the new vaccine and drugs are in evaluation stage. Experiments were conducted on cotton rats and mice in which RSV F specific nano-bodies and immunoglobulin were administered by intranasal route. This led to reduction in lung inflammation and also decreased the virus replication after RSV infection [57]. The RSV G protein is also being targeted for the development of drugs, prophylactic agents and vaccines. The RSV G protein consists of CX3C motif and is homologous in structure with CX3CL1 [58]. RSV G protein increases the infection rate by binding the receptor CX3CR1. Experiments have shown that anti- RSV G monoclonal antibodies have the ability to block the interaction between RSV G CX3C-CX3CR1. This interaction inhibition decreased the lung inflammation. Experiments conducted on rats also have been shown that RSV G monoclonal antibodies have the greater ability to decrease the pulmonary inflammation when compared with anti-F monoclonal antibodies [59–61].

6. Current status of RSV vaccine

At present, there is no approved vaccine is present in the market which can protect from RSV infection. Due to increased burden of disease, it is essential to develop a vaccine that can give protection against the disease [47]. Recently, a lot of RSV vaccine candidates have been emerged using a variety of advanced technologies. About 60 RSV vaccines candidates targeting the pediatric and older populations are in development stage and some are also in preclinical stage [62]. According to a study, 16 RSV vaccine candidates are in clinical development stage [62].

6.1 Live attenuated vaccine

During 1960s, after the failure of formalin inactivated RSV vaccine (FI-RSV), struggles were started to develop live-attenuated vaccines candidates. By serial passaging of RSV A2 strain at lower temperature, live attenuated vaccines were produced; however, it was hard to achieve the balance between immunogenicity and safety [62].

Today, a lot of the cold passage (cp) and temperature sensitive (ts) vaccines have been produced. Evaluation of one cpts-248/404 was done in 1–2 month old aged infants. But it led to the problem such as congestion of upper respiratory tract and so, it was not followed for more investigations. After this struggles were done to attenuate the cpts-248/404 strain and many mutants were produced. After evaluation these generated mutants were found to be over or under attenuated [63].

There is another live-attenuated type RSV vaccine which includes M-2 gene deletion is being tested on nonhuman primates. The M-2 gene regulates the transition from transcription to RNA replication. Studies have shown that by the deletion of M-2 gene, viral RNA replication is decreased but at the same time G and F protein expression is increased through transcription which means that virus is attenuated at adequate level and may lead to neutralizing antibody response [64].

NS2 is another target gene for producing live attenuated vaccine RSV NS2. gene increases the shedding of epithelial cells and reduces or inhibits the antiviral cellular type 1 IFN induction and IFN response of the host. Vaccines which include the deletion of NS2 gene are stable genetically and sensitive to temperature to some extent [65, 66]. SH gene also has been considered for deletion for the live attenuated vaccines. It is believed that SH gene is involved in viral fusion. According to few studies, it is involved in the inhibition of apoptosis by blocking the TNF- alpha pathway. To obtain the sufficient attenuation level to get the safety is the major continuing problem for live attenuated RSV vaccine [65–67].

6.2 Subunit vaccines

RSV G and F glycoproteins lead to the induction of neutralizing antibodies. These have been evaluated as potential vaccine candidate [68]. Subunit vaccines have the potential to be used for maternal immunization. They are also useful candidates for elderly immunization. A number of subunit vaccines have been evaluated recently. The vaccines which are in clinical trials are co-purified G, F and M proteins; purified F glycoprotein (PFP-1, PFP-2 and PFP-3); and BBG2NA etc. [69–76].

RSV PFP-1, PFP-2 and PFP-3 are the candidates which have been evaluated in children of >12 months of age and also in elderly target populations. These vaccine candidates consist of purified glycoprotein which are adsorbed to $Al(OH)_3$ (PFP-1 and PFP-2) or $AlPO_4$ (PFP-3). These candidates were sufficiently tolerated by the target populations but acute reactions were also observed up-to minimum level. There was no observation of enhanced disease occurrence [70–77].

7. Challenges to RSV vaccine development

7.1 Early age when immature immune system of neonates

The most noteworthy risk group for extreme RSV infection is infants under a half year of age [78, 79]. Practically speaking, first dose should be administered at the age of 2 months. Full term newborn children obtain maternal antibodies during the latter 50% of gestation and levels of antibody remain moderately high for a half year after the birth [80]. This would interfere when RSV vaccine would be done [81]. So there is need of an ideal vaccine which will not interfere with the maternal antibodies and will give protection in the presence of maternal antibodies. A few investigations show that newborn children under the age of 8 months have a less serum counter acting agent (antibody) response to characteristic RSV disease as compared to elder ones [82]. A less developed immune system may be the reason of this reduced immunity level, but maternal antibodies may also suppress the immune response [83].

Recent schedule for hepatitis B, diphtheria, rotavirus, pneumococcus, pertussis, tetanus, *Haemophilus influenzae* type b and poliovirus show that vaccine for these infectious diseases will be done ideally after birth at 2, 4 and 6 months of age. Vaccination for RSV should be ideally administered at 6 months of age, so it is necessary and important to make sure that RSV vaccine should not interfere the working and efficacy of other routinely used vaccines during the childhood [84].

7.2 Induction of low affinity neutralizing antibodies

RSV vaccine was developed shortly after it was isolated. In 1960, FI-RSV vaccine was injected by intramuscular route in 2–7 months old infants and children. Instead of providing protection against wild type RSV infection, FI-RSV enhanced the respiratory disease development following wild type RSV infection during the subsequent RSV season. Lungs of children and infants with enhanced diseased were rich with large numbers of eosinophils and this was not found in patients of natural infection with RSV. After this disastrous outcome, there was need to develop a safe RSV vaccine including the evaluation of enhanced disease [47–49, 85, 86].

These different immunopathology aspects which were seen in humans after FI-RSV vaccine and enhanced disease were later studied in non-human primates. In newborn macaques which were FI-RSV vaccinated and then infected with RSV virus, enhanced disease with increased level of eosinophils and neutrophils were seen [87–91]. FI-RSV produced the increased level of ELISA titer RSV antibody because it was highly immunogenic, but the provoked antibodies were non-neutralizing. Antibodies produced did not provide the protection against virus because it could not prevent the fusion of virus [92, 93]. FI-RSV induced resulted RSV antibodies were also known to be of decreased avidity and this may be the result of having lack of maturation [94–97].

7.3 Lack of appropriate animal models

No ideal animal model for RSV vaccine is present which can be used for its evaluation. African green monkey kidney cells (Vero cells) were used for production of RSV. High titers of RSV were observed on Vero cell line. Similar results were obtained when grown on human cells (HEp-2). On both these cell lines, RSV infection led to syncytia formation. These cell lines were used extensively to characterize the live attenuated RSV vaccines. In recent studies, there are reports that NHBE (normal human bronchial epithelial) and HAE (human airway epithelial) cells are used to create model human nasopharyngeal mucosa. RSV infection did not show any pathological sign and also not led to syncytia formation on NHBE and HAE cell lines [98, 99].

Experiments to study attenuation of live attenuated RSV vaccine were also conducted on BALB/c mice, found permissive to infection to some extent. Advantages for mouse studies are that reagents are readily available which can be used for measurement of infection immune correlates [99–104]. Several non-human primates act as host for RSV. RSV can replicate in the nasopharyngeal tract of their host. Macaques, African green monkeys, Chimpanzees and bonnet monkeys have been used to model RSV infection [105–112]. Relative viral titers of live attenuated RSV vaccines compared to wild type RSV disease can also be measured. Chimpanzees are the only non-human hosts which develop and show the clinical sign and symptoms of coryza following RSV infection. They are much permissive to RSV infection. So they are used for evaluation of comparative level of attenuation among vaccines which are candidates in humans. But it has been shown by the recent studies that chimpanzee is not completely predictive of attenuation in young newborns. They are also scare and expensive. Study conducted by Karron et al. showed that those RSV vaccines sensitive to temperature and also had high degree attenuation in chimpanzee, were able to produce infection in lower respiratory tract in children [112].

7.4 Absence of RSV disease liability data and commercial risk

It is known that those children and persons primed with RSV are not at risk to RSV enhanced illness, but the absence of enhanced disease illness in RSV primed persons does not support the prediction that it will not be present in RSV naïve population. So it is very difficult to build up safety data which can support and be used for testation of novel RSV vaccine in newborns having age <6 month which is primary target population [113, 114]. There is absence of information (data) on RSV related mortality. This has prevented exact appraisal of the expenses and advantages of RSV vaccines and prioritization of vaccines for various target populaces [49]. Lack of information on disease liability data is a big problem in less developed countries where mortality cases are concentrated [115].

7.5 Limited resources

Clinical investigations of applicant vaccines in the target populace are fundamental to figure out which vaccines ought to be created for licensure, yet these examinations are tedious and costly, what's more, assets for these investigations are restricted. Measurement of impact of vaccine on disease in all target populations is very difficult and problematic. It is easy to diagnose RSV infection in infants and children because their respiratory secretions have high titers of RSV and so are easy to detect. Titers of virus in adults are low and sensitive RT-PCR assay is used for detection purpose. If there is a decrease in severity of disease, it is a good indication of vaccine being effective. Measures done for disease severity are not accurate at all ages of target populations. So there is need that larger and most costly studies should be performed [116].

7.6 Emerging RSV variants/mutation in RSV genome

RSV is divided antigenically into two groups which are RSV-A and RSV-B. These groups are further divided into genotypes as well as variants. It has been investigated that different viruses belong to these different groups; genotypes as well as variants co-circulate in epidemics. So it is very difficult to develop an effective vaccine due to the presence of virus antigenic diversity as well as variability. Like other RNA viruses, RSV has high nucleotide substitution rate (10^{-3}–10^{-4}). Spontaneous type of deletions of G and SH genes have been studied *in vitro*. RSV genome encodes 11 proteins; one of them is G protein which is most variable having 2 hypervariable regions. G protein has been investigated to accumulate amino acid changes periodically. RSV genotypes having the amino acids duplications in G proteins also have been isolated.

7.7 Disruption of antigenic epitopes

Researches had shown that formalin inactivation caused the alterations in the epitopes of the G and F proteins and as a result non-neutralizing antibodies were developed which led to formation of immune complex in the lungs [57, 69]. Recent studies have shown that changes in the properties of F protein occur during interaction of virus and host cell. The pre fusion (pre-F) which is highly energetic, transitions irreversibly into post fusion (post-F) form which is low energetic and stable, this occurs during insertion process of virus into host cell membrane. By this process, fusion of virus to host occurs. Although pre and post F are not structurally similar, they share 2 antigenic regions. Neutralizing antibodies target these antigenic regions. Pre F also has 3 other antigenic sites not present in post-F. These sites are neutralization sensitive [68–72]. It is investigated that pre-F conformation changes to post-F conformation during the mechanism of formalin as well as heat inactivation and this change is irreversible. As a result of this change, complete loss of epitopes occurs. So this process explains the one of the reasons for failure of FI-RSV [69, 71].

7.8 Older age when immune-senescence of the elderly people

Elder target population group possess a considerable disease burden. The elder group has preexisting immunity, which makes it inconvenient to increase the existing immunity. Furthermore immune-senescence may lead to decrease in the efficacy of vaccine [116]. Immune-senescence is a challenge for proper vaccination in older target populations. RSV disease burden increases in elderly people in presence of underlying diseases such as cardiac and pulmonary conditions. Live attenuated vaccines are found not to be immunogenic in elderly people. So now focus is on subunit vaccines for this target group [115, 117].

8. Future horizons in RSV vaccine and RSV therapeutics

- Continuous struggles are going on for the development of effective and safe RSV vaccines for each target group (infants, children, elders including pregnant women). Previous struggles made to build up a safe vaccine were failed. High antibody production was seen by the use of FI-RSV vaccine in 1960. However, unfortunately vaccinated children developed a severe disease after administration of FI-RSV vaccine. Difficulties and barriers associated with vaccine development particularly live attenuated vaccine are enhanced respiratory disease, maternal antibodies, nasal congestion, low immunogenicity, genetic variability and instability, immature immune system of infants, vaccine virus transmission and immune-senescence as well as preexisting immunity in elders. However, these problems are being slowly overcome [118].

- Major achievements in last 3 years are that nanoparticle based vaccines and live vector vaccines have been investigated in different phase 1 and phase 2 trials and efficient results obtained. These vaccines step forward into later phase trials for evaluation [119]. So, there is hope that safe and well tolerated vaccine candidates will provide a long lasting immunity to all target groups, may be in our hands with in ~5–10 years.

- *In vitro* tissue culture system has been developed, that are being used for predicting the efficacy and safety of candidate vaccines.

- Palivizumab is only the success which is available to clinicians and is being used to reduce the burden of RSV. Palivizumab has decreased hospitalization; however, its use is limited due to high cost. There is hope that this approved prophylactic approach will be available to everyone and may soon come into extensive and widespread use. Palivizumab is patent of MedImmune and this patent is near to expire. So with expiry of this patent, there is hope that a cost effective palivizumab version will be developed. A recent technology hub has been established by the World Health Organization (WHO), the purpose of this is to increase the production of biosimilar versions [120]. There is hope that these products will be available in the market at low and affordable cost. These good initiatives will greatly reduce the mortality rates caused by RSV in developing world.

- Oral antivirals such as GS-5806 and a nucleoside analogue ALS-008176 have been passed through trials and they significantly decreased the replication of virus in human controlled experiments [121]. Nanobodies (single domain antibodies) has also been developed that protected the mice from infection and now are ready for clinical development. These results renewed the hope that an effective antiviral treatment for different risk populace will be on the horizon in next few years [57].

9. Conclusions

One of the most common causes of the respiratory tract diseases is the RSV affecting infants, young children and the elderly people. Only supportive treatment is available such as corticosteroids, bronchodilators, oxygen supplement and ribavirin etc. which may not be occasionally effective. Palivizumab has decreased hospitalization; however, its use is limited due to high cost. Despite it is the era of progress and technology, no RSV licensed vaccine is available in the market to prevent RSV infection. Natural infection also provides partial immunity. A successful vaccine candidate will provide the long term protective immunity and must not lead to induction of enhanced RSV disease. For RSV vaccine development different target groups are being considered such as elders including pregnant women, children and infants. Each of these target groups has different challenges for vaccine development. Maternal antibodies, enhanced disease and immature immune system are the major barriers for vaccine development in the infants. The children >6 months of age have more mature immune system than infants but still can be at the risk of enhanced disease from non-live RSV vaccine. For elderly target population immune-senescence as well as pre-existing immunity is the barrier for vaccine development.

An ideal RSV vaccine should be safe, well tolerated and provide long lasting immunity as compared to natural infection against both RSV strains A and

B. Further, it is recommended that separate vaccines should be developed for each target group. The tools that ought to enable us to build up a sheltered and successful RSV vaccine are accessible and our challenge is to utilize them wisely. We trust the suggestions for vaccine advancement noted above can support researchers, subsidizing offices, and industry center their endeavors and assets most productively and viably.

Conflict of interest

There is no potential conflict of interest among the authors listed in this manuscript.

Author details

Muhammad Shafique[1]*, Muhammad Asif Zahoor[1], Muhammad Imran Arshad[2], Bilal Aslam[1], Abu Baker Siddique[1], Muhammad Hidayat Rasool[1], Muhammad Usman Qamar[1] and Muhammad Usman[1]

1 Department of Microbiology, Government College University, Faisalabad, Pakistan

2 Institute of Microbiology, University of Agriculture Faisalabad, Pakistan

*Address all correspondence to: drmshafique@gcuf.edu.pk

References

[1] Dowell SF, Anderson LJ, Gary HE Jr, Erdman DD, Plouffe JF, File TM Jr, et al. Respiratory syncytial virus is an important cause of community-acquired lower respiratory infection among hospitalized adults. The Journal of Infectious Diseases. 1996;**174**(3):456-462

[2] Falsey AR, Hennessey PA, Formica MA, Cox C, Walsh EE. Respiratory syncytial virus infection in elderly and high-risk adults. The New England Journal of Medicine. 2005;**352**(17):1749-1759

[3] Null DM, Bimle C, Weisman LE, Johnson K, Steichen J, Singh S, et al. Palivizumab, a humanized respiratory syncytial virus monoclonal antibody, reduces hospitalization from respiratory syncytial virus infection in high-risk infants. Pediatrics. 1998;**102**(3 Pt 1): 531-537

[4] Vandini S, Biagi C, Lanari M. Respiratory syncytial virus: The influence of serotype and genotype variability on clinical course of infection. International Journal of Molecular Sciences. 2017; **18**(8):pii.E1717. DOI: 10.3390/ijms18081717

[5] Hacking D, Hull J. Respiratory syncytial virus—Viral biology and the host response. The Journal of Infection. 2002;**45**(1):18-24

[6] Shafique M, Rasool MH, Khurshid M. Respiratory syncytial virus: An overview of infection biology and vaccination strategies. Future Virology. 2017;**12**(5):297-313

[7] Spann KM, Tran KC, Collins PL Effects of nonstructural proteins NS1 and NS2 of human respiratory syncytial virus on interferon regulatory factor 3, NF-kappaB, and proinflammatory cytokines. Journal of Virology. 2005;**79**(9):5353-5362

[8] Feldman SA, Audet S, Beeler JA. The fusion glycoprotein of human respiratory syncytial virus facilitates virus attachment and infectivity via an interaction with cellular heparan sulfate. Journal of Virology. 2000;**74**(14):6442-6447

[9] Feldman SA, Crim RL, Audet SA, Beeler JA. Human respiratory syncytial virus surface glycoproteins F, G and SH form an oligomeric complex. Archives of Virology. 2001;**146**(12):2369-2383

[10] Gonzalez PA, Bueno SM, Carreno LJ, Riedel CA, Kalergis AM. Respiratory syncytial virus infection and immunity. Reviews in Medical Virology. 2012;**22**(4):230-244

[11] Cheng X, Park H, Zhou H, Jin H. Overexpression of the M2-2 protein of respiratory syncytial virus inhibits viral replication. Journal of Virology. 2005;**79**(22):13943-13952

[12] Fearns R, Collins PL. Role of the M2-1 transcription antitermination protein of respiratory syncytial virus in sequential transcription. Journal of Virology. 1999;**73**(7):5852-5864

[13] Spence L, Barratt N. Respiratory syncytial virus associated with acute respiratory infections in Trinidadian patients. American Journal of Epidemiology. 1968;**88**(2):257-266

[14] Huq F, Rahman M, Nahar N, Alam A, Haque M, Sack DA, et al. Acute lower respiratory tract infection due to virus among hospitalized children in Dhaka, Bangladesh. Reviews of Infectious Diseases. 1990;**12**(Suppl 8): S982-S987

[15] Vardas E, Blaauw D, McAnerney J. The epidemiology of respiratory syncytial virus (RSV) infections in South African children. South African Medical Journal. 1999;**89**(10):1079-1084

[16] Byrd LG, Prince GA. Animal models of respiratory syncytial virus infection. Clinical Infectious Diseases. 1997;**25**(6):1363-1368

[17] Hall CB, Douglas RG Jr. Modes of transmission of respiratory syncytial virus. The Journal of Pediatrics. 1981;**99**(1):100-103

[18] Henderson FW, Collier AM, Clyde WA Jr, Denny FW. Respiratory-syncytial-virus infections, reinfections and immunity. A prospective, longitudinal study in young children. The New England Journal of Medicine. 1979;**300**(10):530-534

[19] Hall CB, Walsh EE, Long CE, Schnabel KC. Immunity to and frequency of reinfection with respiratory syncytial virus. The Journal of Infectious Diseases. 1991;**163**(4):693-698

[20] Reed G, Jewett PH, Thompson J, Tollefson S, Wright PF. Epidemiology and clinical impact of parainfluenza virus infections in otherwise healthy infants and young children <5 years old. The Journal of Infectious Diseases. 1997;**175**(4):807-813

[21] Shay DK, Holman RC, Newman RD, Liu LL, Stout JW, Anderson LJ. Bronchiolitis-associated hospitalizations among US children, 1980-1996. JAMA. 1999;**282**(15):1440-1446

[22] Tissing WJ, van Steensel-Moll HA, Offringa M. Risk factors for mechanical ventilation in respiratory syncytial virus infection. European Journal of Pediatrics. 1993;**152**(2):125-127

[23] Green M, Brayer AF, Schenkman KA, Wald ER. Duration of hospitalization in previously well infants with respiratory syncytial virus infection. The Pediatric Infectious Disease Journal. 1989;**8**(9):601-605

[24] Navas L, Wang E, de Carvalho V, Robinson J. Improved outcome of respiratory syncytial virus infection in a high-risk hospitalized population of Canadian children. Pediatric Investigators Collaborative Network on Infections in Canada. The Journal of Pediatrics. 1992;**121**(3):348-354

[25] Groothuis JR, Gutierrez KM, Lauer BA. Respiratory syncytial virus infection in children with bronchopulmonary dysplasia. Pediatrics. 1988;**82**(2):199-203

[26] MacDonald NE, Hall CB, Suffin SC, Alexson C, Harris PJ, Manning JA. Respiratory syncytial viral infection in infants with congenital heart disease. The New England Journal of Medicine. 1982;**307**(7):397-400

[27] Hall CB, Powell KR, MacDonald NE, Gala CL, Menegus ME, Suffin SC, et al. Respiratory syncytial viral infection in children with compromised immune function. The New England Journal of Medicine. 1986;**315**(2):77-81

[28] Welliver RC. Review of epidemiology and clinical risk factors for severe respiratory syncytial virus (RSV) infection. The Journal of Pediatrics. 2003;**143**(5 Suppl):S112-S117

[29] Hall CB, Long CE, Schnabel KC. Respiratory syncytial virus infections in previously healthy working adults. Clinical Infectious Diseases. 2001;**33**(6):792-796

[30] Han LL, Alexander JP, Anderson LJ. Respiratory syncytial virus pneumonia among the elderly: an assessment of disease burden. The Journal of Infectious Diseases. 1999;**179**(1):25-30

[31] Falsey AR, Walsh EE. Respiratory syncytial virus infection in adults. Clinical Microbiology Reviews. 2000;**13**(3):371-384

[32] Hall WJ, Hall CB, Speers DM. Respiratory syncytial virus infection in adults: clinical, virologic, and serial pulmonary function studies. Annals of Internal Medicine. 1978;**88**(2):203-205

[33] Miyairi I, DeVincenzo JP. Human genetic factors and respiratory syncytial virus disease severity. Clinical Microbiology Reviews. 2008;**21**(4):686-703

[34] Culley FJ, Pennycook AM, Tregoning JS, Hussell T, Openshaw PJ. Differential chemokine expression following respiratory virus infection reflects Th1- or Th2-biased immunopathology. Journal of Virology. 2006;**80**(9):4521-4527

[35] Garofalo RP, Patti J, Hintz KA, Hill V, Ogra PL, Welliver RC. Macrophage inflammatory protein-1alpha (not T helper type 2 cytokines) is associated with severe forms of respiratory syncytial virus bronchiolitis. The Journal of Infectious Diseases. 2001;**184**(4):393-399

[36] Parrott RH, Kim HW, Arrobio JO, Hodes DS, Murphy BR, Brandt CD, et al. Epidemiology of respiratory syncytial virus infection in Washington, D.C. II. Infection and disease with respect to age, immunologic status, race and sex. American Journal of Epidemiology. 1973;**98**(4):289-300

[37] Brandenburg AH, Jeannet PY, Steensel-Moll HA, Ott A, Rothbarth PH, Wunderli W, et al. Local variability in respiratory syncytial virus disease severity. Archives of Disease in Childhood. 1997;**77**(5):410-414

[38] Singleton RJ, Petersen KM, Berner JE, Schulte E, Chiu K, Lilly CM, et al. Hospitalizations for respiratory syncytial virus infection in Alaska Native children. The Pediatric Infectious Disease Journal. 1995;**14**(1):26-30

[39] McConnochie KM, Roghmann KJ. Breast feeding and maternal smoking as predictors of wheezing in children age 6 to 10 years. Pediatric Pulmonology. 1986;**2**(5):260-268

[40] Wright AL, Holberg C, Martinez FD, Taussig LM. Relationship of parental smoking to wheezing and nonwheezing lower respiratory tract illnesses in infancy. Group Health Medical Associates. The Journal of Pediatrics. 1991;**118**(2):207-214

[41] Jung JW. Respiratory syncytial virus infection in children with congenital heart disease: Global data and interim results of Korean RSV-CHD survey. Korean Journal of Pediatrics. 2011;**54**(5):192-196

[42] Walsh EE, McConnochie KM, Long CE, Hall CB. Severity of respiratory syncytial virus infection is related to virus strain. The Journal of Infectious Diseases. 1997;**175**(4):814-820

[43] Hornsleth A, Klug B, Nir M, Johansen J, Hansen KS, Christensen LS, et al. Severity of respiratory syncytial virus disease related to type and genotype of virus and to cytokine values in nasopharyngeal secretions. The Pediatric Infectious Disease Journal. 1998;**17**(12):1114-1121

[44] Devincenzo JP. Natural infection of infants with respiratory syncytial virus subgroups A and B: A study of frequency, disease severity, and viral load. Pediatric Research. 2004;**56**(6):914-917

[45] DeVincenzo JP, El Saleeby CM, Bush AJ. Respiratory syncytial virus load predicts disease severity in previously healthy infants. The Journal of Infectious Diseases. 2005;**191**(11):1861-1868

[46] van Drunen Littel-van den Hurk S, Mapletoft JW, Arsic N, Kovacs-Nolan J. Immunopathology of RSV infection: Prospects for developing

vaccines without this complication. Reviews in Medical Virology. 2007;**17**(1):5-34

[47] Kim HW, Canchola JG, Brandt CD, Pyles G, Chanock RM, Jensen K, et al. Respiratory syncytial virus disease in infants despite prior administration of antigenic inactivated vaccine. American Journal of Epidemiology. 1969;**89**(4):422-434

[48] Fulginiti VA, Eller JJ, Sieber OF, Joyner JW, Minamitani M, Meiklejohn G. Respiratory virus immunization. I. A field trial of two inactivated respiratory virus vaccines; an aqueous trivalent parainfluenza virus vaccine and an alum-precipitated respiratory syncytial virus vaccine. American Journal of Epidemiology. 1969;**89**(4):435-448

[49] Chin J, Magoffin RL, Shearer LA, Schieble JH, Lennette EH. Field evaluation of a respiratory syncytial virus vaccine and a trivalent parainfluenza virus vaccine in a pediatric population. American Journal of Epidemiology. 1969;**89**(4):449-463

[50] Roymans D, Koul A. Treatment of respiratory syncytial virus infection: Past, present and future. In: Resch B, editor. Human Respiratory Syncytial Virus Infection. Rijeka, Croatia: In Tech; 2011. pp. 197-215

[51] Patel H, Platt R, Lozano JM, Wang EE. Glucocorticoids for acute viral bronchiolitis in infants and young children. Cochrane Database of Systematic Reviews. 2008;**1**:CD004878

[52] Kellner JD, Ohlsson A, Gadomski AM, Wang EE. Bronchodilators for bronchiolitis. Cochrane Database of Systematic Reviews. 2006;**3**:CD001266

[53] Ventre K, Randolph A. Ribavirin for respiratory syncytial virus infection of the lower respiratory tract in infants and young children. Cochrane Database of Systematic Reviews. 2007;**1**:CD000181

[54] Rezaee F, Linfield DT, Harford TJ, Piedimonte G. Ongoing developments in RSV prophylaxis: A clinician's analysis. Current Opinion in Virology. 2017;**24**:70-78

[55] Dawson-Caswell M, Muncie HL Jr. Respiratory syncytial virus infection in children. American Family Physician. 2011;**83**(2):141-146

[56] Turner TL, Kopp BT, Paul G, et al. Respiratory syncytial virus: Current and emerging treatment options. ClinicoEconomics and Outcomes Research. 2014;**6**:217-225

[57] Schepens B, Ibañez LI, De Baets S, et al. Nanobodies specific for respiratory syncytial virus fusion protein protect against infection by inhibition of fusion. The Journal of Infectious Diseases. 2011;**204**:1692-1701

[58] Tripp RA, Jones LP, Haynes LM, Zheng H, Murphy PM, Anderson LJ. CX3C chemokine mimicry by respiratory syncytial virus G glycoprotein. Nature Immunology. 2001;**2**:732-738

[59] Haynes LM, Caidi H, Radu GU, et al. Therapeutic monoclonal antibody treatment targeting respiratory syncytial virus (RSV) G protein mediates viral clearance and reduces the pathogenesis of RSV infection in BALB/c mice. The Journal of Infectious Diseases. 2009;**200**:439-447

[60] Kauvar LM, Harcourt JL, Haynes LM, Tripp RA. Therapeutic targeting of respiratory syncytial virus G-protein. Immunotherapy. 2010;**2**:655-661

[61] Caidi H, Harcourt JL, Tripp RA, Anderson LJ, Haynes LM. The effects of combination therapy using monoclonal antibodies against RSV G glycoprotein in BALB/c mice. PLoS ONE. 2012;**7**: e51485

[62] Deboarh H, Carrie T, Cheryl K. Advances in RSV vaccine research and

development: A global agenda. Vaccine. 2016;**34**:2870-2875

[63] Gonzalez IM, Karron RA, Eichelberger M, et al. Evaluation of the live attenuated cpts 248/404 RSV vaccine in combination with a subunit RSV vaccine (PFP-2) in healthy young and older adults. Vaccine. 2000;**18**:1763-1772

[64] Teng MN, Whitehead SS, Bermingham A, et al. Recombinant respiratory syncytial virus that does not express the NS1or M2-2 protein is highly attenuated and immunogenic in chimpanzees. Journal of Virology. 2000;**74**:9317-9321

[65] Luongo C, Winter CC, Collins PL, Buchholz UJ. Respiratory syncytial virus modified by deletions of the NS2 gene and amino acid S1313 of the L polymerase protein is a temperature-sensitive, live-attenuated vaccine candidate that is phenotypically stable at physiological temperature. Journal of Virology. 2013;**87**:1985-1996

[66] Liesman RM, Buchholz UJ, Luongo CL, Yang L, Proia AD, DeVincenzo JP, et al. RSV-encoded NS2 promotes epithelial cell shedding and distal airway obstruction. The Journal of Clinical Investigation. 2014;**124**:2219-2233

[67] Cunningham CK. R. A Phase I study of the safety and immunogenicity of a single dose of the recombinant live attenuated respiratory syncytial virus vaccine RSV cps2, Lot RSV#005A, Delivered as nose drops to RSV-seronegative infants and children 6 to 24 months of age. Edited by: Regulatory compliance and human subjects protection branch (RCHSPB), Division of clinical research (DCR)/Office of the director (OD), The national institute of allergy and infectious diseases (NIAID), The eunice kennedy shriver national institute of child health and Human development (NICHD); 2013. pp. 10-20

[68] Collins PL, Chanock RM, Murphy BR. Respiratory syncytial virus. In: Knipe DM, Howley PM, Griffin DE, et al., editors. Fields Virology. 4th ed. Vol. 1. Philadelphia: Lippincott Williams & Wilkins; 2001. pp. 1443-1485

[69] Falsey AR, Walsh EE. Safety and immunogenicity of a respiratory syncytial virus subunit vaccine (PFP 2) in ambulatory adults over age 60. Vaccine. 1996;**14**:1214-1218

[70] Falsey AR, Walsh EE. Safety and immunogenicity of a respiratory syncytial virus subunit vaccine (PFP-2) in the institutionalized elderly. Vaccine. 1997;**15**:1130-1132

[71] Belshe RB, Anderson EL, Walsh EE. Immunogenicity of purified F glycoprotein of respiratory syncytial virus: Clinical and immune responses to subsequent natural infection in children. The Journal of Infectious Diseases. 1993;**168**:1024-1029

[72] Paradiso PR, Hildreth SW, Hogerman DA, et al. Safety and immunogenicity of a subunit respiratory syncytial virus vaccine in children 24 to 48 months old. The Pediatric Infectious Disease Journal. 1994;**13**:792-798

[73] Tristram DA, Welliver RC, Mohar CK, Hogerman DA, Hildreth SW, Paradiso P. Immunogenicity and safety of respiratory syncytial virus subunit vaccine in seropositive children 18-36 months old. The Journal of Infectious Diseases. 1993;**167**:191-195

[74] Piedra PA, Grace S, Jewell A, et al. Purified fusion protein vaccine protects against lower respiratory tract illness during respiratory syncytial virus season in children with cystic fibrosis. The Pediatric Infectious Disease Journal. 1996;**15**:23-31

[75] Groothuis JR, King SJ, Hogerman DA, Paradiso PR, Simoes EA. Safety and immunogenicity of a purified F

protein respiratory syncytial virus (PFP-2) vaccine in seropositive children with bronchopulmonary dysplasia. The Journal of Infectious Diseases. 1998;**177**:467-469

[76] Munoz FM, Piedra PA, Maccato M, Kozinetz C, Glezen WP. Respiratory syncytial virus purified fusion protein-2 (RSV-PFP-2) vaccine in pregnancy [abstract]. In: RSV After 45 Years. Segovia, Spain: Instituto de Salud Carlos, Ministerio de Sanidad y Consumo; 2001. p. 45

[77] Power UF, Plotnicky-Gilquin H, Huss T, et al. Induction of protective immunity in rodents by vaccination with a prokaryotically expressed recombinant fusion protein containing a respiratory syncytial virus G protein fragment. Virology. 1997;**230**: 155-166

[78] Lee M-S, Walker RE, Mendelman PM. Medical burden of respiratory syncytial virus and parainfluenza virus type 3 infection among US children, implications for design of vaccine trials. Human Vaccines. 2005;**1**:6-11

[79] Karron RA, Singelton RJ, Bulkow L, Parkinson A, Kruse D, De Smet I, et al. Severe respiratory syncytial virus disease in Alaska native children. The Journal of Infectious Diseases. 1999;**180**:41-49

[80] Brandenburg AH, Groen J, van Steensel-Moll HA, Claas ECJ, Rothbarth PH, Neijens HJ, et al. Respiratory syncytial virus specific serum antibodies in infants under six months of age: limited serological response upon infection. Journal of Medical Virology. 1997;**52**:97-104

[81] Groothuis JR, Simoes E, Myron JL, Hall CB, Long CE, Rodriguez WJ, et al. Prophylactic administration of respiratory syncytial virus immune globulin to high-risk infants and young children. The New England Journal of Medicine. 1993;**329**:1524-1530

[82] Centers for Disease Control and Prevention. Recommended immunization schedule for persons aged 0-6 years. United States: 2008; www.cdc.gov/vaccines/recs/schedules

[83] Hall CB, Weinberg GA, Iwane MK, Blumkin AK, Edwards KM, Staat MA, et al. The burden of respiratory syncytial virus infection in young children. The New England Journal of Medicine. 2009;**360**:588-598

[84] Nair H, Nokes DJ, Gessner BD, Dherani M, Madhi SA, Singleton RJ, et al. Global burden of acute lower respiratory infections due to respiratory syncytial virus in young children: A systematic review and meta-analysis. Lancet. 2010;**375**:1545-1555

[85] Kapikian AZ, Mitchell RH, Chanock RM, Shvedoff RA, Stewart CE. An epidemiologic study of altered clinical reactivity to respiratory syncytial (RS) virus infection in children previously vaccinated with an inactivated RSV virus vaccine. American Journal of Epidemiology. 1969;**89**:405-421

[86] Kim HW, Arrobio JO, Pyles G, Brandt CD, Camargo E, Chanock RM, et al. Clinical and immunological response of infants and children to administration of low-temperature adapted respiratory syncytial virus. Pediatrics. 1971;**48**:745-755

[87] Prince GA, Jensen BA, Hemming VG. Enhancement of respiratory syncytial virus pulmonary pathology in cotton rats by prior intramuscular inoculation of formalin-inactivated virus. Journal of Virology. 1986;**57**:721-728

[88] De Swart RL, Kuiken T, Timmerman HH, Van Amerongen G, Van Den Hoogen BG, Vos HW, et al. Immunization of macaques with

formalin-inactivated respiratory syncytial virus (RSV) induces interleukin-13-associatedhypersensitivity to subsequent RSV infection. Journal of Virology. 2002;**76**:11561-11569

[89] Polack FP, Teng MN, Collins PL, Prince GA, Exner M, Regele H, et al. A role for immune complexes in enhanced respiratory syncytial virus disease. The Journal of Experimental Medicine. 2002;**196**:859-865

[90] Polack FR. A typical measles and enhanced respiratory syncytial virus disease (ERD) made simple. Pediatric Research. 2007;**62**:111-115

[91] Waris ME, Tsou C, Erdman DD, Zaki WR, Anderson LJ. Respiratory syncytial virus infection in BALB/c mice previously immunized with formalin-inactivated virus induces enhance pulmonary inflammatory response with a predominant Th2-like cytokine pattern. Journal of Virology. 1996;**70**:2852-2860

[92] Murphy BR, Walsh EE. Formalin-inactivated respiratory syncytial virus vaccine induces antibodies to the fusion glycoprotein that are deficient in fusion-inhibiting activity. Journal of Clinical Microbiology. 1988;**26**:1595-1597

[93] Moghaddam A, Olszewska W, Wang B, Tregoning JS, Helson R, Sattentau Q J, et al. A potential molecular mechanism for hypersensitivity caused by formalin-inactivated vaccines. Nature Medicine. 2006;**12**:905-907

[94] Delgado MF, Coviello S, Monsalvo AC, Melendi GA, Hernandez JZ, Batalle JP, et al. Lack of antibody affinity maturation due to poor Toll-like receptor stimulation leads to enhanced respiratory syncytial virus disease. Nature Medicine. 2008;**15**:34-41

[95] Wright PF, Karron RA, Belshe RB, Shi JR, Randolph VB, Collins PL, et al. The absence of enhanced disease with wild type respiratory syncytial virus infection occurring after receipt of live, attenuated, respiratory syncytial virus vaccines. Vaccine. 2007;**25**:7372-7378

[96] Murphy BR, Collins PL. Live-attenuated virus vaccines for respiratory syncytial and parainfluenza viruses: Applications of reverse genetic. The Journal of Clinical Investigation. 2002;**110**:21-27

[97] Murphy BR, Hall SL, Kulkarni AB, Crowe JE Jr, Collins PL, Connors M, et al. An update on approaches to the development of respiratory syncytial virus (RSV) and parainfluenza virus type 3 (PIV3) vaccines. Virus Research. 1994;**32**:13-36

[98] Wright PF, Ikizler MR, Gonzales RA, Carroll KN, Johnson JE, Werkhaven JA. Growth of respiratory syncytial virus in primary epithelial cells from the human respiratory tract. Journal of Virology. 2005;**79**:8651-8654

[99] Zhang L, Peeples ME, Boucher RC, Collins PL, Pickles RJ. Respiratory syncytial virus infection of human airway epithelial cells is polarized, specific to ciliated cells, and without obvious cytopathology. Journal of Virology. 2002;**76**:5654-5666

[100] Jafri HS, Chavez-Bueno S, Mejias A, Rios AM, Shahryar SN, Usuf M, et al. Respiratory syncytial virus lower respiratory tract infection induces acute pneumonia, cytokine response, airway obstruction and chronic inflammatory infiltrates associated with longterm airway hyper-responsiveness in mice. The Journal of Infectious Diseases. 2004;**189**:1856-1865

[101] Mejais A, Cavez-Bueno S, Rios AM, Saavedra-Lozano J, Aten MF, Hatfield J, et al. Anti-respiratory syncytial virus (RSV) neutralizing antibody decreases lung inflammation, airway obstruction, and airway hyper-responsiveness in a murine RSV model. Antimicrobial

Agents and Chemotherapy. 2004;**48**: 1811-1822

[102] Prince GA, Horswood RL, Camargo E, Koenig D, Chanock RM. Mechanisms of immunity to respiratory syncytial virus in cotton rats. Infection and Immunity. 1983;**42**:81-87

[103] Prince GA, Prieels J-P, Slaoui M, Porter DD. Pulmonary lesions in primary respiratory syncytial virus infection, reinfection, and vaccine-enhanced disease in the cotton rat (*Sigmodon hispidus*). Laboratory Investigation. 1999;**79**:1385-1392

[104] Blanco JC, Richardson JY, Narnell ME, Rowzee A, Pletneva L, Porter DD, et al. Cytokine and chemokine gene expresssion after primary and secondary respiratory syncytial virus infection in cotton rats. The Journal of Infectious Diseases. 2002;**185**:1780-1785

[105] Crowe JE Jr, Bui PT, Davis AR, Chanock RM, Murphy BR. A further attenuated derivative of a cold passaged temperature-sensitive mutant of human respiratory syncytial virus retains immunogenicity and protective efficacy against wild-type challenge in seronegative chimpanzees. Vaccine. 1994;**12**:783-790

[106] Hsu KHL, Lubeck MD, Davis AR, Bhat RA, Selling BH, Bhat BM, et al. Immunogenicity of recombinant adenovirus-respiratory syncytial virus using Ad4, Ad5, Ad7 vectors in dogs and a chimpanzee. The Journal of Infectious Diseases. 1992;**166**:766-769

[107] Jin H, Cheng X, Train-Dorge VL, Park HJ, Zhou H, Soike K, et al. Evaluation of recombinant respiratory syncytial virus gene deletion mutants in African green monkeys for their potential as live attenuated vaccine candidates. Vaccine. 2003;**21**:3647-3652

[108] Simoes EA, Hayward AR, Ponnuraj EM, Straumanis JP, Stenmark KR, Wilson HL, et al. Respiratory syncytial virus infects the Bonnet monkey, Macaca radiata. Pediatric and Developmental Pathology. 1999;**2**: 316-326

[109] Teng MN, Whithehead SS, Bermingham A, St. Claire M, Elkins WR, Murphy BR, et al. Recombinant respiratory syncytial virus that does not express the NS1 or M2-2 protein is highly attenuated and immunogenic in chimpanzees. Journal of Virology. 2000;**74**:9317-9321

[110] Whitehead SS, Bukreyev A, Teng MN, Firestone C-Y, St. Claire M, Elkins WR, et al. Recombinant respiratory syncytial virus bearing a deletion of either the NS2 or SH gene is attenuated in chimpanzees. Journal of Virology. 1999;**73**:3438-3442

[111] Whitehead SS, Juhasz K, Firestone C-Y, Collins PL, Murphy BR. Recombinant respiratory syncytial virus (RSV) bearing a set of mutations from cold-passaged RSV is attenuated in chimpanzees. Journal of Virology. 1998;**72**:4467-4471

[112] Karron RA, Wright PF, Crowe JE, Clements-Mann ML, Thompson J, Makhene M, et al. Evaluation of two live, cold-passaged, temperature-sensitive respiratory syncytial virus vaccines in chimpanzees and in human adults, infants and children. The Journal of Infectious Diseases. 1997;**176**:1428-1436

[113] Graham BS. Biological challenges and technological opportunities for respiratory syncytial virus vaccine development. Immunological Reviews. 2011;**239**:149-166

[114] Shay DK, Holman RC, Newman RD, Liu LL, Stout JW, Anderson LJ. Bronchiolitis-associated hospitalizations among U.S. children, 1980-1995. The Journal of the American Medical Association. 1999;**282**:1440-1447

[115] Acedo L, Diez-Domingo J, Morano JA, Villanueva RJ. Mathematical modelling of respiratory syncytial virus (RSV): vaccination strategies and budget applications. Epidemiology and Infection. 2010;**138**:853-860

[116] Anderson LJ, Dormitzerb PR, Nokesc DJ, Rappuolie DR, Roca A, Graham BS. Strategic priorities for respiratory syncytial virus (RSV) vaccine development. Vaccine. 2013;**31S**:B209-B215

[117] Stockman LJ, Curns AT, Anderson LJ, Fischer-Langley G. Respiratory syncytial virus-associated hospitalizations among infants and young children in the United States, 1997-2006. The Pediatric Infectious Disease Journal. 2012;**31**:5-9

[118] Green C, Scarselli E, Sande C, Thompson A, De Lara C, Taylor K, et al. Chimpanzee adenovirusand MVA-vectored respiratory syncytial virus vaccine is safe and immunogenic in adults. Science Translational Medicine. 2015;7:300ra126

[119] Glenn G, Smith G, Fries L, Raghunandan R, Lu H, Zhou B, et al. Safety and immunogenicity of a Sf9 insect cell-derived respiratory syncytial virus fusion protein nanoparticle vaccine. Vaccine. 2013;**31**:524-532

[120] Humphreys G. Hubs to spread technology and save lives. Bulletin of the World Health Organization. 2015;**93**:290-291

[121] DeVincenzo J, Fathi H, McClure M, Westland C, Chanda S, Lambkin-Williams R, et al. Treatment with oral ALS-008176, a nucleoside analog, rapidly reduces RSV viral load and clinical disease severity in a healthy volunteer challenge study. Open Forum Infectious Diseases. 2014;**1**(Suppl. 1): S66-S69